R for Health Data Science

T0179500

R for Health Data Science

Ewen Harrison
Riinu Pius

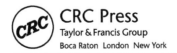

CRC Press
Taylor & Francis Group
Boca Raton London New York

CRC Press is an imprint of the
Taylor & Francis Group, an **informa** business

A CHAPMAN & HALL BOOK

First edition published 2021
by CRC Press
6000 Broken Sound Parkway NW, Suite 300, Boca Raton, FL 33487-2742

and by CRC Press
2 Park Square, Milton Park, Abingdon, Oxon, OX14 4RN

ISBN: 9780367428327 (hbk)
ISBN: 9780367428198 (pbk)
ISBN: 9780367855420 (ebk)

Typeset in Computer Modern font
by KnowledgeWorks Global Ltd.

"The future is already here — it's just not evenly distributed."

William Gibson

Contents

Preface

Why read this book

> We are drowning in information but starved for knowledge.
> John Naisbitt

In this age of information, the manipulation, analysis and interpretation of data have become a fundamental part of professional life. Nowhere more so than in the delivery of healthcare. From the understanding of disease and the development of new treatments, to the diagnosis and management of individual patients, the use of data and technology are now an integral part of the business of healthcare.

Those working in healthcare interact daily with data, often without realising it. The conversion of this avalanche of information to useful knowledge is essential for high-quality patient care. An important part of this information revolution is the opportunity for everybody to become involved in data analysis. This democratisation is driven in part by the open source software movement – no longer do we require expensive specialised software to do this.

The statistical programming language, R, is firmly at the heart of this.

This book will take an individual with little or no experience in data science all the way through to the execution of sophisticated analyses. We emphasise the importance of truly understanding the underlying data with liberal use of plotting, rather than relying on opaque and possibly poorly understood statistical tests. There are numerous examples included that can be adapted for your own data, together with our own R packages with easy-to-use functions.

We have a lot of fun teaching this course and focus on making the material as accessible as possible. We limit equations to a minimum in favour of code, and use examples rather than lengthy explanations. We are grateful to the many individuals and students who have helped refine this book and welcome suggestions and bug reports via `https://github.com/SurgicalInformatics`.

Ewen Harrison and Riinu Pius

Usher Institute

University of Edinburgh

Contributors

We are indebted to the following people who have generously contributed time and material to this book: Katie Connor, Tom Drake, Cameron Fairfield, Peter Hall, Stephen Knight, Kenneth McLean, Lisa Norman, Einar Pius, Michael Ramage, Katie Shaw, and Olivia Swann.

About the Authors

Ewen Harrison is a surgeon and Riinu Pius is a physicist. And they're both data scientists, too. They dabble in a few programming languages and are generally all over technology. They are most enthusiastic about the R statistical programming language and have a combined experience of 25 years using it. They work at the University of Edinburgh and have taught R to hundreds of healthcare professionals and researchers.

They believe a first introduction to R and statistical programming should be relatively jargon-free and outcome-oriented (get those pretty plots out). The understanding of complicated concepts will come over time with practice and experience, not through a re-telling of the history of computing bit-by-byte, or with the inclusion of the underlying equations for each statistical test (although Ewen has sneaked a few equations in).

Overall, they hope to make the text fun and accessible. Just like them.

Part I

Data wrangling and visualisation

1

Why we love R

Thank you for choosing this book on using R for health data analysis. Even if you're already familiar with the R language, we hope you will find some new approaches here as we make the most of the latest R tools including some we've developed ourselves. Those already familiar with R are encouraged to still skim through the first few chapters to familiarise yourself with the style of R we recommend.

R can be used for all the health data science applications we can think of. From bioinformatics and computational biology, to administrative data analysis and natural language processing, through internet-of-things and wearable data, to machine learning and artificial intelligence, and even public health and epidemiology. R has it all.

Here are the main reasons we love R:

- R is versatile and powerful - use it for
  - graphics;
  - all the statistical tests you can dream of;
  - machine learning and deep learning;
  - automated reports;
  - websites;
  - and even books (yes, this book was written entirely in R).
- R scripts can be reused - gives you efficiency and reproducibility.
- It is free to use by anyone, anywhere.

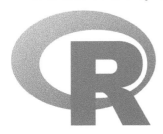

1.1   Help, what's a script?

A script is a list of instructions. It is just a text file and no special software is required to view one. An example R script is shown in Figure 1.1.

Don't panic! The only thing you need to understand at this point is that what you're looking at is a list of instructions written in the R language.

You should also notice that some parts of the script look like normal English. These are the lines that start with a # and they are called "comments". We can (and should) include these comments in everything we do. These are notes of what we were doing, both for colleagues as well as our future selves.

```
example_script.R ✕
                        Source on Save   🔍  ⚗ ▾  ☐
 1   # Loading two packages into your library
 2   # tidyverse and gapminder
 3   library(tidyverse)
 4   library(gapminder)
 5
 6   # Modify data
 7   gapminder2007 = gapminder %>%
 8     filter(year == 2007)
 9
10   # Plot data
11   gapminder2007 %>%
12     ggplot(aes(x = gdpPercap, y = lifeExp)) +
13     geom_point()
14
15   # Statistical test
16   t.test(lifeExp ~ gdpPercap > 20000, data = gapminder2007)
17
18
```

FIGURE 1.1: An example R script from RStudio.

Lines that do not start with # are R code. This is where the number crunching really happens. We will cover the details of this R code in the next few chapters. The purpose of this chapter is to describe some of the terminology as well as the interface and tools we use.

For the impatient:

- We interface R using RStudio

- We use the **tidyverse** packages that are a substantial extension to base R functionality (we repeat: extension, not replacement)

Even though R is a language, don't think that after reading this book you should be able to open a blank file and just start typing in R code like an evil computer genius from a movie. This is not what real-world programming looks like.

Firstly, you should be copy-pasting and adapting existing R code examples - whether from this book, the internet, or later from your existing work. Re-writing everything from scratch is not efficient. Yes, you will understand and eventually remember a lot of it, but to spend time memorising specific functions that can easily be looked up and copied is simply not necessary.

Secondly, R is an interactive language. Meaning that we "run" R code line by line and get immediate feedback. We do not write a whole script without trying each part out as we go along.

Thirdly, do not worry about making mistakes. Celebrate them! The whole point of R and reproducibility is that manipulations are not applied directly on a dataset, but a copy of it. Everything is in a script, so you can't do anything wrong. If you make a mistake like accidentally overwriting your data, we can just reload it, rerun the steps that worked well and continue figuring out what went wrong at the end. And since all of these steps are written down in a script, R will redo everything with a single push of a button. You do not have to repeat a set of mouse clicks from dropdown menus as in other statistical packages, which quickly becomes a blessing.

1.2 What is RStudio?

RStudio is a free program that makes working with R easier. An example screenshot of RStudio is shown in Figure 1.2. We have already introduced what is in the top-left pane - the **Script**.

Now, look at the little **Run** and **Source** buttons at the top-right corner of the script pane. Clicking **Run** executes a line of R code. Clicking **Source** executes all lines of R code in the script (it is essentially 'Run all lines'). When you run R code, it gets sent to the **Console** which is the bottom-left panel. This is where R really lives.

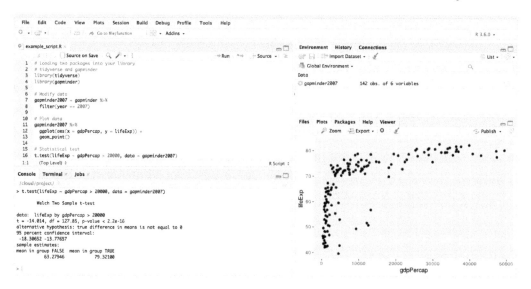

FIGURE 1.2: We use RStudio to work with R.

Keyboard Shortcuts!
Run line: Control+Enter
Run all lines (Source): Control+Shift+Enter
(On a Mac, both Control or Command work)

The Console is where R speaks to us. When we're lucky, we get results in there - in this example the results of a *t*-test (last line of the script). When we're less lucky, this is also where Errors or Warnings appear.

R Errors are a lot less scary than they seem! Yes, if you're using a regular computer program where all you do is click on some buttons, then getting a proper red error that stops everything is quite unusual. But in programming, Errors are just a way for R to communicate with us.

We see Errors in our own work every single day, they are very normal and do not mean that everything is wrong or that you should give up. Try to re-frame the word Error to mean "feedback", as in "Hello, this is R. I can't continue, this is the feedback I am giving you." The most common Errors you'll see are along the lines of "Error: something not found". This almost always means there's a typo or you've misspelled something. Furthermore, R is case sensitive so capitalisation matters (variable name `lifeExp` is not the same as `lifeexp`).

The Console can only print text, so any plots you create in your script appear in the **Plots** pane (bottom-right).

Similarly, datasets that you've loaded or created appear in the **Environment** tab. When you click on a dataset, it pops up in a nice viewer that is fast even when there is a lot of data. This means you can have a look and scroll through your rows and columns, the same way you would with a spreadsheet.

1.3   Getting started

To start using R, you should do these two things:

- Install R (from `https://www.r-project.org/`)
- Install RStudio Desktop (from `https://www.rstudio.com/`)

When you first open up RStudio, you'll also want to install some extra packages to extend the base R functionality. You can do this in the **Packages** tab (next to the Plots tab in the bottom-right in Figure 1.2).

A Package is just a collection of functions (commands) that are not included in the standard R installation, called base-R.

A lot of the functionality introduced in this book comes from the **tidyverse** family of R packages (`http://tidyverse.org` Wickham et al. (2019)). So when you go to Packages, click **Install**, type in **tidyverse**, and a whole collection of useful and modern packages will be installed.

Even though you've installed the **tidyverse** packages, you'll still need to tell R when you're about to use them. We include `library(tidyverse)` at the top of every script we write:

```
library(tidyverse)

Registered S3 methods overwritten by 'dbplyr':
  method             from
  print.tbl_lazy
  print.tbl_sql
— Attaching packages ————— tidyverse 1.3.0 —
✓ ggplot2 3.3.2       ✓ purrr    0.3.4
✓ tibble  3.0.3       ✓ dplyr    1.0.0
✓ tidyr   1.1.0       ✓ stringr 1.4.0
✓ readr   1.3.1       ✓ forcats 0.5.0
— Conflicts ————————— tidyverse_conflicts() —
x dplyr::filter() masks stats::filter()
x dplyr::lag()    masks stats::lag()
```

We can see that it has loaded 8 packages (**ggplot2, tibble, tidyr, readr,**

purrr, **dplyr**, **stringr**, **forcats**), the number behind a package name is its version.

The "Conflicts" message is expected and can safely be ignored.[1]

There are a few other R packages that we use and are not part of the tidyverse, but we will introduce them as we go along. If you're incredibly curious, head to the Resources section of the HealthyR website which is the best place to find up-to-date links and installation instructions. Our R and package versions are also listed in the Appendix.

1.4   Getting help

The best way to troubleshoot R errors is to copy-paste them into a search engine (e.g., Google). Searching online is also a great way to learn how to do new specific things or to find code examples. You should copy-paste solutions into your R script to then modify to match what you're trying to do. We are constantly copying code from online forums and our own existing scripts.

However, there are many different ways to achieve the same thing in R. Sometimes you'll search for help and come across R code that looks nothing like what you've seen in this book. The **tidyverse** packages are relatively new and use the pipe (`%>%`), something we'll come on to. But search engines will often prioritise older results that use a more traditional approach.

So older solutions may come up at the top. Don't get discouraged if you see R code that looks completely different to what you were expecting. Just keep scrolling down or clicking through different answers until you find something that looks a little bit more familiar.

If you're working offline, then RStudio's built in **Help** tab is useful. To use the Help tab, click your cursor on something in your code (e.g., `read_csv()`) and press F1. This will show you the definition and some examples. F1 can be hard to find on some keyboards, an alternative is to type, e.g., `?read_csv`. This will also open the Help tab for this function.

---

[1]It just means that when we use `filter` or `lag`, they will come from the **dplyr** package, rather than the **stats** package. We've never needed to use `filter` and `lag` from **stats**, but if you do, then use the double colon, i.e., `stats::filter()` or `stats::lag()`, as just `filter()` will use the **dplyr** one.

However, the Help tab is only useful if you already know what you are looking for but can't remember exactly how it works. For finding help on things you have not used before, it is best to Google it.

R has about 2 million users so someone somewhere has probably had the same question or problem.

RStudio also has a Help drop-down menu at the very top (same row where you find "File", "Edit", ...). The most notable things in the Help drop-down menu are the Cheatsheets. These tightly packed two-pagers include many of the most useful functions from tidyverse packages. They are not particularly easy to learn from, but invaluable as an *aide-mémoire*.

1.5 Work in a Project

The files on your computer are organised into folders. RStudio Projects live in your computer's normal folders - they placemark the working directory of each analysis project. These project folders can be viewed or moved around the same way you normally work with files and folders on your computer.

The top-right corner of your RStudio should never say **"Project: (None)"**. If it does, click on it and create a New Project. After clicking on New Project, you can decide whether to let RStudio create a New Directory (folder) on your computer. Alternatively, if your data files are already organised into an "Existing folder", use the latter option.

Every set of analysis you are working on must have its own folder and RStudio project. This enables you to switch between different projects without getting the data, scripts, or output files all mixed up. Everything gets read in or saved to the correct place. No more exporting a plot and then going through the various Documents, etc., folders on your computer trying to figure out where your plot might have been saved to. It got saved to the project folder.

1.6 Restart R regularly

Have you tried turning it off and on again? It is vital to restart R regularly. Restarting R helps to avoid accidentally using the wrong data or functions stored in the environment. Restarting R only takes a second and we do it several times per day! Once you get used to saving everything in a script, you'll always be happy to restart R. This will help you develop robust and reproducible data analysis skills.

You can restart R by clicking on Session -> Restart R (top menu).

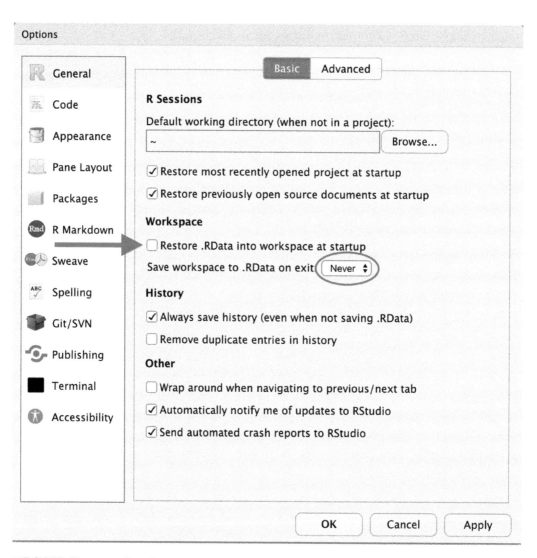

FIGURE 1.3: Configuring your RStudio Tools -> Global Options: Untick "Restore .RData into Workspace on Exit" and Set "Save .RData on exit" to Never.

Furthermore, RStudio has a default setting that is no longer considered best practice (Figure 1.3). After installing RStudio, you should go change two small but important things in `Tools -> Global Options`:

1. **Uncheck** "Restore .RData into Workspace on startup"
2. Set "Save .RData on exit" to **Never**

This does not mean you can't or shouldn't save your work in `.RData/.rda` files. But it is best to do it consciously and load exactly what you want to load. Letting R silently save and load everything for you may also include broken data or objects.

1.7 Notation throughout this book

When mentioned in the text, the names of R packages are in bold font, e.g., **ggplot2**, whereas functions, objects, and variables are printed with mono-spaced font, e.g `filter()`, `mean()`, `lifeExp`. Functions are always followed by brackets: `()`, whereas data objects or variables are not.

Otherwise, R code lives in the grey areas known as 'code chunks'. Lines of R *output* start with a double ## - this will be the numbers or text that R gives us after executing code. R also adds a counter at the beginning of every new line; look at the numbers in the square brackets [] below:

```
# colon between two numbers creates a sequence
1001:1017
```

```
##  [1] 1001 1002 1003 1004 1005 1006 1007 1008 1009 1010 1011 1012 1013 1014 1015
## [16] 1016 1017
```

Remember, lines of R code that start with # are called comments. We already introduced comments as notes about the R code earlier in this chapter (Section 1.1 "Help, what's a script?"), however, there is a second use case for comments.

When you make R code a comment, by adding a # in front of it, it gets 'commented out'. For example, let's say your R script does two things, prints numbers from 1 to 4, and then numbers from 1001 to 1004:

```
# Let's print small numbers:
1:4
```

```
## [1] 1 2 3 4
```

```
# Now we're printing bigger numbers:
1001:1004
```

```
## [1] 1001 1002 1003 1004
```

If you decide to 'comment out' the printing of big numbers, the code will look like this:

```
# Let's print small numbers:
1:4
```

```
# Now we're printing bigger numbers:
# 1001:1004
```

```
## [1] 1 2 3 4
```

You may even want to add another real comment to explain why the latter was commented out:

```
# Now commented out as not required any more
# Now we're printing bigger numbers:
# 1001:1004
```

You could of course delete the line altogether, but commenting out is useful as you might want to include the lines later by removing the # from the beginning of the line.

Keyboard Shortcut for commenting out/commenting in multiple lines at a time: Control+Shift+C
(On a Mac, both Control or Command work)

2

R basics

Throughout this book, we are conscious of the balance between theory and practice. Some learners may prefer to see all definitions laid out before being shown an example of a new concept. Others would rather see practical examples and explanations build up to a full understanding over time. We strike a balance between these two approaches that works well for most people in the audience.

Sometimes we will show you an example that may use words that have not been formally introduced yet. For example, we start this chapter with data import - R is nothing without data.

In so doing, we have to use the word "argument", which is only defined two sections later (in 2.3 "Objects and functions"). A few similar instances arise around statistical concepts in the Data Analysis part of the book. You will come across sentences along the lines of "this concept will become clearer in the next section". Trust us and just go with it.

The aim of this chapter is to familiarise you with how R works. We will read in data and start basic manipulations. You may want to skip parts of this chapter if you already:

- have found the Import Dataset interface;
- know what numbers, characters, factors, and dates look like in R;
- are familiar with the terminology around objects, functions, arguments;
- have used the pipe: `%>%`;
- know how to filter data with operators such as `==`, `>`, `<`, `&`, `|`;
- know how to handle missing data (NAs), and why they can behave weirdly in a filter;
- have used `mutate()`, `c()`, `paste()`, `if_else()`, and the joins.

2.1   Reading data into R

Data usually comes in the form of a table, such as a spreadsheet or database. In the world of the **tidyverse**, a table read into R gets called a `tibble`.

A common format in which to receive data is CSV (comma separated values). CSV is an uncomplicated spreadsheet with no formatting. It is just a single table with rows and columns (no worksheets or formulas). Furthermore, you don't need special software to quickly view a CSV file - a text editor will do, and that includes RStudio.

For example, look at "example_data.csv" in the healthyr project's folder in Figure 2.1 (this is the Files pane at the bottom-right corner of your RStudio).

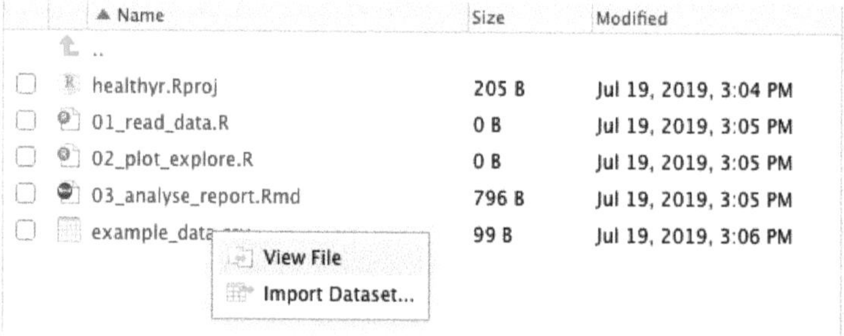

FIGURE 2.1: View or import a data file.

Clicking on a data file gives us two options: "View File" or "Import Dataset".

We will show you how to use the Import Dataset interface in a bit, but for standard CSV files, we don't usually bother with the Import interface and just type in (or copy from a previous script):

```
library(tidyverse)
example_data <- read_csv("example_data.csv")
View(example_data)
```

There are a couple of things to say about the first R code chunk of this book. First and foremost: do not panic. Yes, if you're used to interacting with data by double-clicking on a spreadsheet that just opens up, then the above R code does seem a bit involved.

However, running the example above also has an immediate visual effect. As soon as you click Run (or press Ctrl+Enter/Command+Enter), the dataset immediately shows up in your Environment and opens in a Viewer. You can have a look and scroll through the same way you would in Excel or similar.

So what's actually going on in the R code above:

- We load the **tidyverse** packages (as covered in the first chapter of this book).
- We have a CSV file called "example_data.csv" and are using `read_csv()` to read it into R.
- We are using the assignment arrow `<-` to save it into our Environment using the same name: `example_data`.
- The `View(example_data)` line makes it pop up for us to view it. Alternatively, click on `example_data` in the Environment to achieve the exact same thing.

More about the assignment arrow (`<-`) and naming things in R are covered later in this chapter. Do not worry if everything is not crystal clear just now.

2.1.1   Import Dataset interface

In the `read_csv()` example above, we read in a file that was in a specific (but common) format.

However, if your file uses semicolons instead of commas, or commas instead of dots, or a special number for missing values (e.g., 99), or anything else weird or complicated, then we need a different approach.

RStudio's **Import Dataset** interface (Figure 2.1) can handle all of these and more.

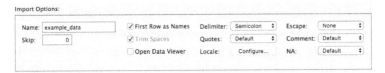

FIGURE 2.2: Import: Some of the special settings your data file might have.

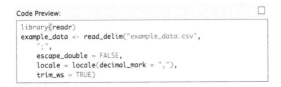

FIGURE 2.3: After using the Import Dataset window, copy-paste the resulting code into your script.

After selecting the specific options to import a particular file, a friendly preview window will show whether R properly understands the format of your data.

DO NOT BE tempted to press the **Import** button.

Yes, this will read in your dataset once, but means you have to reselect the options every time you come back to RStudio. Instead, copy-paste the code (e.g., Figure 2.3) into your R script. This way you can use it over and over again.

Ensuring that all steps of an analysis are recorded in scripts makes your workflow reproducible by your future self, colleagues, supervisors, and extraterrestrials.

The `Import Dataset` button can also help you to read in Excel, SPSS, Stata, or SAS files (instead of `read_csv()`, it will give you `read_excel()`, `read_sav()`, `read_stata()`, or `read_sas()`).

If you've used R before or are using older scripts passed by colleagues, you might see `read.csv()` rather than `read_csv()`. Note the dot rather than the underscore.

In short, `read_csv()` is faster and more predictable and in all new scripts is to be recommended.

In existing scripts that work and are tested, we do not recommend that you start replacing `read.csv()` with `read_csv()`. For instance, `read_csv()` handles categorical variables differently [1]. An R script written using the `read.csv()` might not work as expected any more if just replaced with `read_csv()`.

Do not start updating and possibly breaking existing R scripts by replacing base R functions with the tidyverse equivalents we show here. Do use the modern functions in any new code you write.

2.1.2 Reading in the Global Burden of Disease example dataset

In the next few chapters of this book, we will be using the Global Burden of Disease datasets. The Global Burden of Disease Study (GBD) is the most comprehensive worldwide observational epidemiological study to date. It de-

---

[1]It does not silently convert strings to factors, i.e., it defaults to `stringsAsFactors = FALSE`. For those not familiar with the terminology here - don't worry, we will cover this in just a few sections.

scribes mortality and morbidity from major diseases, injuries and risk factors to health at global, national and regional levels. [2]

GBD data are publicly available from the website. Table 2.1 and Figure 2.4 show a high level version of the project data with just 3 variables: cause, year, deaths_millions (number of people who die of each cause every year). Later, we will be using a longer dataset with different subgroups and we will show you how to summarise comprehensive datasets yourself.

```
library(tidyverse)
gbd_short <- read_csv("data/global_burden_disease_cause-year.csv")
```

TABLE 2.1: Deaths per year from three broad disease categories (short version of the Global Burden of Disease example dataset).

year	cause	deaths_millions
1990	Communicable diseases	15.36
1990	Injuries	4.25
1990	Non-communicable diseases	26.71
1995	Communicable diseases	15.11
1995	Injuries	4.53
1995	Non-communicable diseases	29.27
2000	Communicable diseases	14.81
2000	Injuries	4.56
2000	Non-communicable diseases	31.01
2005	Communicable diseases	13.89
2005	Injuries	4.49
2005	Non-communicable diseases	32.87
2010	Communicable diseases	12.51
2010	Injuries	4.69
2010	Non-communicable diseases	35.43
2015	Communicable diseases	10.88
2015	Injuries	4.46
2015	Non-communicable diseases	39.28
2017	Communicable diseases	10.38
2017	Injuries	4.47
2017	Non-communicable diseases	40.89

2.2 Variable types and why we care

There are three broad types of data:

---

[2] Global Burden of Disease Collaborative Network. Global Burden of Disease Study 2017 (GBD 2017) Results. Seattle, United States: Institute for Health Metrics and Evaluation (IHME), 2018. Available from http://ghdx.healthdata.org/gbd-results-tool.

A

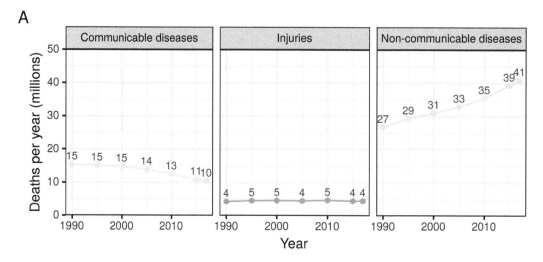

B

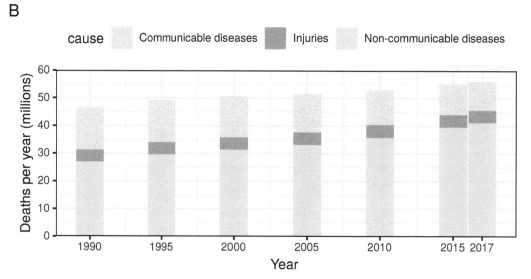

FIGURE 2.4: Line and bar charts: Cause of death by year (GBD). Data in (B) are the same as (A) but stacked to show the total of all causes.

- continuous (numbers), in R: numeric, double, or integer;
- categorical, in R: character, factor, or logical (TRUE/FALSE);
- date/time, in R: POSIXct date-time[3].

Values within a column all have to be the same type, but a tibble can of course hold columns of different types. Generally, R is good at figuring out what type of data you have (in programming, this 'figuring out' is called 'parsing').

---

[3]Portable Operating System Interface (POSIX) is a set of computing standards. There's nothing more to understand about this other than when R starts shouting "POSIXct this or POSIXlt that" at you, check your date and time variables

For example, when reading in data, it will tell you what was assumed for each column:

```
library(tidyverse)
typesdata <- read_csv("data/typesdata.csv")
```

```
## Parsed with column specification:
## cols(
##    id = col_character(),
##    group = col_character(),
##    measurement = col_double(),
##    date = col_datetime(format = "")
## )
```

```
typesdata
```

```
## # A tibble: 3 x 4
##    id    group       measurement date
##    <chr> <chr>             <dbl> <dttm>
## 1 ID1   Control             1.8 2017-01-02 12:00:00
## 2 ID2   Treatment           4.5 2018-02-03 13:00:00
## 3 ID3   Treatment           3.7 2019-03-04 14:00:00
```

This means that a lot of the time you do not have to worry about those little <chr> vs <dbl> vs <S3: POSIXct> labels. But in cases of irregular or faulty input data, or when doing a lot of calculations and modifications to your data, we need to be aware of these different types to be able to find and fix mistakes.

For example, consider a similar file as above but with some data entry issues introduced:

```
typesdata_faulty <- read_csv("data/typesdata_faulty.csv")
```

```
## Parsed with column specification:
## cols(
##    id = col_character(),
##    group = col_character(),
##    measurement = col_character(),
##    date = col_character()
## )
```

```
typesdata_faulty
```

```
## # A tibble: 3 x 4
##    id    group     measurement date
##    <chr> <chr>     <chr>       <chr>
## 1 ID1   Control   1.8         02-Jan-17 12:00
## 2 ID2   Treatment 4.5         03-Feb-18 13:00
## 3 ID3   Treatment 3.7 or 3.8  04-Mar-19 14:00
```

Notice that R parsed both the measurement and date variables as characters. Measurement has been parsed as a character because of a data entry issue: the person taking the measurement couldn't decide which value to note down (maybe the scale was shifting between the two values) so they included both values and text "or" in the cell.

A numeric variable will also get parsed as a categorical variable if it contains certain typos, e.g., if entered as "3..7" instead of "3.7".

The reason R didn't automatically make sense of the date column is that it couldn't tell which is the date and which is the year: `02-Jan-17` could stand for `02-Jan-2017` as well as `2002-Jan-17`.

Therefore, while a lot of the time you do not have to worry about variable types and can just get on with your analysis, it is important to understand what the different types are to be ready to deal with them when issues arise.

Since health datasets are generally full of categorical data, it is crucial to understand the difference between characters and factors (both are types of categorical variables in R with pros and cons).

So here we go.

2.2.1   Numeric variables (continuous)

Numbers are straightforward to handle and don't usually cause trouble. R usually refers to numbers as `numeric` (or `num`), but sometimes it really gets its nerd on and calls numbers `integer` or `double`. Integers are numbers without decimal places (e.g., `1`, `2`, `3`), whereas `double` stands for "Double-precision floating-point" format (e.g., `1.234`, `5.67890`).

It doesn't usually matter whether R is classifying your continuous data `numeric/num/double/int`, but it is good to be aware of these different terms as you will see them in R messages.

Something to note about numbers is that R doesn't usually print more than 6 decimal places, but that doesn't mean they don't exist. For example, from the `typedata` tibble, we're taking the `measurement` column and sending it to the `mean()` function. R then calculates the mean and tells us what it is with 6 decimal places:

```
typesdata$measurement %>% mean()
```

```
## [1] 3.333333
```

Let's save that in a new object:

```
measurement_mean <- typesdata$measurement %>% mean()
```

But when using the double equals operator to check if this is equivalent to a fixed value (you might do this when comparing to a threshold, or even another mean value), R returns FALSE:

```
measurement_mean == 3.333333
```

```
## [1] FALSE
```

Now this doesn't seem right, does it - R clearly told us just above that the mean of this variable is 3.333333 (reminder: the actual values in the measurement column are 1.8, 4.5, 3.7). The reason the above statement is FALSE is because measurement_mean is quietly holding more than 6 decimal places.

And it gets worse. In this example, you may recognise that repeating decimals (0.333333...) usually mean there's more of them somewhere. And you may think that rounding them down with the round() function would make your == behave as expected. Except, it's not about rounding, it's about how computers store numbers with decimals. Computers have issues with decimal numbers, and this simple example illustrates one:

```
(0.10 + 0.05) == 0.15
```

```
## [1] FALSE
```

This returns FALSE, meaning R does not seem to think that 0.10 + 0.05 is equal to 0.15. This issue isn't specific to R, but to programming languages in general. For example, python also thinks that the sum of 0.10 and 0.05 does not equal 0.15.

This is where the near() function comes in handy:

```
library(tidyverse)
near(0.10+0.05, 0.15)
```

```
## [1] TRUE
```

```
near(measurement_mean, 3.333333, 0.000001)
```

```
## [1] TRUE
```

The first two arguments for `near()` are the numbers you are comparing; the third argument is the precision you are interested in. So if the numbers are equal within that precision, it returns TRUE. You can omit the third argument - the precision (in this case also known as the tolerance). If you do, `near()` will use a reasonable default tolerance value.

2.2.2 Character variables

Characters (sometimes referred to as *strings* or *character strings*) in R are letters, words, or even whole sentences (an example of this may be free text comments). Characters are displayed in-between "" (or ' ').

A useful function for quickly investigating categorical variables is the `count()` function:

```
library(tidyverse)
typesdata %>%
  count(group)
```

```
## # A tibble: 2 x 2
##    group        n
##    <chr>    <int>
## 1 Control      1
## 2 Treatment    2
```

`count()` can accept multiple variables and will count up the number of observations in each subgroup, e.g., `mydata %>% count(var1, var2)`.

Another helpful option to count is `sort = TRUE`, which will order the result putting the highest count (`n`) to the top.

```
typesdata %>%
  count(group, sort = TRUE)
```

```
## # A tibble: 2 x 2
##    group        n
##    <chr>    <int>
## 1 Treatment    2
## 2 Control      1
```

`count()` with the `sort = TRUE` option is also useful for identifying duplicate IDs or misspellings in your data. With this example `tibble` (`typesdata`) that only has three rows, it is easy to see that the `id` column is a unique identifier whereas the `group` column is a categorical variable.

You can check everything by just eyeballing the `tibble` using the built in Viewer tab (click on the dataset in the Environment tab).

But for larger datasets, you need to know how to check and then clean data programmatically - you can't go through thousands of values checking they are all as intended without unexpected duplicates or typos.

For most variables (categorical or numeric), we recommend always plotting your data before starting analysis. But to check for duplicates in a unique identifier, use `count()` with `sort = TRUE`:

```
# all ids are unique:
typesdata %>%
  count(id, sort = TRUE)
```

```
## # A tibble: 3 x 2
##    id         n
##    <chr> <int>
## 1 ID1        1
## 2 ID2        1
## 3 ID3        1
```

```
# we add in a duplicate row where id = ID3,
# then count again:
typesdata %>%
  add_row(id = "ID3") %>%
  count(id, sort = TRUE)
```

```
## # A tibble: 3 x 2
##    id         n
##    <chr> <int>
## 1 ID3        2
## 2 ID1        1
## 3 ID2        1
```

2.2.3 Factor variables (categorical)

Factors are fussy characters. Factors are fussy because they include something called *levels*. Levels are all the unique values a factor variable could take, e.g., like when we looked at `typesdata %>% count(group)`. Using factors rather than just characters can be useful because:

- The values factor levels can take are fixed. For example, once you tell R that `typesdata$group` is a factor with two levels: Control and Treatment, combining it with other datasets with different spellings or abbreviations for the same variable will generate a warning. This can be helpful but can also be a nuisance when you really do want to add in another level to a `factor` variable.
- Levels have an order. When running statistical tests on grouped data (e.g., Control vs Treatment, Adult vs Child) and the variable is just a character,

not a factor, R will use the alphabetically first as the reference (comparison) level. Converting a character column into a factor column enables us to define and change the order of its levels. Level order affects many things including regression results and plots: by default, categorical variables are ordered alphabetically. If we want a different order in say a bar plot, we need to convert to a factor and reorder before we plot it. The plot will then order the groups correctly.

So overall, since health data is often categorical and has a reference (comparison) level, then factors are an essential way to work with these data in R. Nevertheless, the fussiness of factors can sometimes be unhelpful or even frustrating. A lot more about factor handling will be covered later (8).

2.2.4 Date/time variables

R is good for working with dates. For example, it can calculate the number of days/weeks/months between two dates, or it can be used to find what future date is (e.g., "what's the date exactly 60 days from now?"). It also knows about time zones and is happy to parse dates in pretty much any format - as long as you tell R how your date is formatted (e.g., day before month, month name abbreviated, year in 2 or 4 digits, etc.). Since R displays dates and times between quotes (" "), they look similar to characters. However, it is important to know whether R has understood which of your columns contain date/time information, and which are just normal characters.

```
library(lubridate) # lubridate makes working with dates easier
current_datetime <- Sys.time()
current_datetime
```

```
## [1] "2020-09-15 15:13:02 BST"
```

```
my_datetime <- "2020-12-01 12:00"
my_datetime
```

```
## [1] "2020-12-01 12:00"
```

When printed, the two objects - `current_datetime` and `my_datetime` seem to have a similar format. But if we try to calculate the difference between these two dates, we get an error:

```
my_datetime - current_datetime
```

```
## [1] "Error in `-.POSIXt`(my_datetime, current_datetime)"
```

That's because when we assigned a value to `my_datetime`, R assumed the simpler type for it - so a character. We can check what the type of an object or variable is using the `class()` function:

```
current_datetime %>% class()
```

```
## [1] "POSIXct" "POSIXt"
```

```
my_datetime %>% class()
```

```
## [1] "character"
```

So we need to tell R that `my_datetime` does indeed include date/time information so we can then use it in calculations:

```
my_datetime_converted <- ymd_hm(my_datetime)
my_datetime_converted
```

```
## [1] "2020-12-01 12:00:00 UTC"
```

Calculating the difference will now work:

```
my_datetime_converted - current_datetime
```

```
## Time difference of 76.90761 days
```

Since R knows this is a difference between two date/time objects, it prints them in a nicely readable way. Furthermore, the result has its own type; it is a "difftime".

```
my_datesdiff <- my_datetime_converted - current_datetime
my_datesdiff %>% class()
```

```
## [1] "difftime"
```

This is useful if we want to apply this time difference on another date, e.g.:

```
ymd_hm("2021-01-02 12:00") + my_datesdiff
```

```
## [1] "2021-03-20 09:46:57 UTC"
```

But if we want to use the number of days in a normal calculation, e.g., what if a measurement increased by 560 arbitrary units during this time period. We might want to calculate the increase per day like this:

```
560/my_datesdiff
```

```
## [1] "Error in `/.difftime`(560, my_datesdiff)"
```

Doesn't work, does it. We need to convert `my_datesdiff` (which is a difftime value) into a numeric value by using the `as.numeric()` function:

```
560/as.numeric(my_datesdiff)
```

```
## [1] 7.281465
```

The **lubridate** package comes with several convenient functions for parsing dates, e.g., `ymd()`, `mdy()`, `ymd_hm()`, etc. - for a full list see `lubridate.tidyverse.org`.

However, if your date/time variable comes in an extra special format, then use the `parse_date_time()` function where the second argument specifies the format using the specifiers given in Table 2.2.

TABLE 2.2: Date/time format specifiers.

Notation	Meaning	Example
%d	day as number	01-31
%m	month as number	01-12
%B	month name	January-December
%b	abbreviated month	Jan-Dec
%Y	4-digit year	2019
%y	2-digit year	19
%H	hours	12
%M	minutes	01
%S	seconds	59
%A	weekday	Monday-Sunday
%a	abbreviated weekday	Mon-Sun

For example:

```
parse_date_time("12:34 07/Jan'20", "%H:%M %d/%b'%y")
```

```
## [1] "2020-01-07 12:34:00 UTC"
```

Furthermore, the same date/time specifiers can be used to rearrange your date and time for printing:

```
Sys.time()
```

```
## [1] "2020-09-15 15:13:02 BST"
```

```
Sys.time() %>% format("%H:%M on %B-%d (%Y)")
```

```
## [1] "15:13 on September-15 (2020)"
```

You can even add plain text into the `format()` function, R will know to put the right date/time values where the % are:

TABLE 2.3: Example of data in columns and rows, including missing values denoted NA (Not applicable/Not available). Once this dataset has been read into R it gets called dataframe/tibble.

id	sex	var1	var2	var3
1	Male	4	NA	2
2	Female	1	4	1
3	Female	2	5	NA
4	Male	3	NA	NA

```
Sys.time() %>% format("Happy days, the current time is %H:%M %B-%d (%Y)!")
```

```
## [1] "Happy days, the current time is 15:13 September-15 (2020)!"
```

```
Sys.time() %>% format("Happy days, the current time is %H:%M %B-%d (%Y)!")
```

```
## [1] "Happy days, the current time is 15:13 September-15 (2020)!"
```

2.3 Objects and functions

There are two fundamental concepts in statistical programming that are important to get straight - objects and functions. The most common object you will be working with is a dataset. This is usually something with rows and columns much like the example in Table 2.3.

To get the small and made-up "dataset" into your Environment, copy and run this code[4]:

```
library(tidyverse)
mydata <- tibble(
  id   = 1:4,
  sex  = c("Male", "Female", "Female", "Male"),
  var1 = c(4, 1, 2, 3),
  var2 = c(NA, 4, 5, NA),
  var3 = c(2, 1, NA, NA)
)
```

Data can live anywhere: on paper, in a spreadsheet, in an SQL database, or in your R Environment. We usually initiate and interface with R using RStudio, but everything we talk about here (objects, functions, environment) also work

---

[4]`c()` stands for combine and will be introduced in more detail later in this chapter

when RStudio is not available, but R is. This can be the case if you are working on a supercomputer that can only serve the R Console and not RStudio.

2.3.1   `data frame/tibble`

So, regularly shaped data in rows and columns is called a table when it lives outside R, but once you read/import it into R it gets called a tibble. If you've used R before, or get given a piece of code that uses `read.csv()` instead of `read_csv()`, you'll have come across the term `data frame`.[5]

A `tibble` is the modern/**tidyverse** version of a data frame in R. In most cases, `data frames` and `tibbles` work interchangeably, but `tibbles` often work better. Another great alternative to base R `data frames` are `data tables`. In this book, and for most of our day-to-day work these days, we will use `tibbles`.

2.3.2   Naming objects

When you read data into R, you want it to show up in the Environment tab. Everything in your Environment needs to have a name. You will likely have many objects such as tibbles going on at the same time. Note that tibble is what the thing is, rather than its name. This is the 'class' of an object.

To keep our code examples easy to follow, we call our example tibble `mydata`. In a real analysis, you should give your tibbles meaningful names, e.g., `patient_data`, `lab_results`, `annual_totals`, etc. Object names can't have spaces in it, which is why we use the underscore (_) to separate words. Object names can include numbers, but they can't start with a number: so `labdata2019` works, `2019labdata` does not.

So, the tibble named `mydata` is an example of an object that can be in the Environment of your R Session:

```
mydata
```

```
## # A tibble: 4 x 5
##       id sex      var1  var2  var3
##    <int> <chr>   <dbl> <dbl> <dbl>
## 1     1 Male        4    NA     2
## 2     2 Female      1     4     1
## 3     3 Female      2     5    NA
## 4     4 Male        3    NA    NA
```

---

[5] `read.csv()` comes with base R, whereas `read_csv()` comes from the `readr` package within the `tidyverse`. We recommend using `read_csv()`.

2.3.3 Function and its arguments

A function is a procedure which takes some information (input), does something to it, and passes back the modified information (output).

A simple function that can be applied to numeric data is `mean()`.

R functions always have round brackets after their name. This is for two reasons. First, it easily differentiates them as functions - you will get used to reading them like this.
Second, and more importantly, we can put *arguments* in these brackets.

Arguments can also be thought of as input. In data analysis, the most common input for a function is data. For instance, we need to give `mean()` some data to average over. It does not make sense (nor will it work) to feed `mean()` the whole tibble with multiple columns, including patient IDs and a categorical variable (`sex`).

To quickly extract a single column, we use the `$` symbol like this:

```
mydata$var1
```

```
## [1] 4 1 2 3
```

You can ignore the `## [1]` at the beginning of the extracted values - this is something that becomes more useful when printing multiple lines of data as the number in the square brackets keeps count on how many values we are seeing.

We can then use `mydata$var1` as the first argument of `mean()` by putting it inside its brackets:

```
mean(mydata$var1)
```

```
## [1] 2.5
```

which tells us that the mean of `var1` (4, 1, 2, 3) is 2.5. In this example, `mydata$var1` is the first and only argument to `mean()`.

But what happens if we try to calculate the average value of `var2` (NA, 4, 5, NA) (remember, `NA` stands for Not Applicable/Available and is used to denote missing data):

```
mean(mydata$var2)
```

```
## [1] NA
```

So why does `mean(mydata$var2)` return NA ("not available") rather than the mean of the values included in this column? That is because the column includes missing values (NAs), and R does not want to average over NAs implicitly. It is being cautious - what if you didn't know there were missing values for some patients? If you wanted to compare the means of `var1` and `var2` without any further filtering, you would be comparing samples of different sizes.

We might expect to see an NA if we tried to, for example, calculate the average of `sex`. And this is indeed the case:

```
mean(mydata$sex)
```

```
## Warning in mean.default(mydata$sex): argument is not numeric or logical:
## returning NA
```

```
## [1] NA
```

Furthermore, R also gives us a pretty clear Warning suggesting it can't compute the mean of an argument that is not numeric or logical. The sentence actually reads pretty fun, as if R was saying it was not logical to calculate the mean of something that is not numeric.

But, R is actually saying that it is happy to calculate the mean of two types of variables: numerics or logicals, but what you have passed is neither.

If you decide to ignore the NAs and want to calculate the mean anyway, you can do so by adding this argument to `mean()`:

```
mean(mydata$var2, na.rm = TRUE)
```

```
## [1] 4.5
```

Adding `na.rm = TRUE` tells R that you are happy for it to calculate the mean of any existing values (but to remove - `rm` - the NA values). This 'removal' excludes the NAs from the calculation, it does not affect the actual tibble (`mydata`) holding the dataset.

R is case sensitive, so `na.rm`, not `NA.rm` etc. There is, however, no need to memorize how the arguments of functions are exactly spelled - this is what the Help tab is for (press F1 when the cursor is on the name of the function). Help pages are built into R, so an internet connection is not required for this.

Make sure to separate multiple arguments with commas or R will give you an error of `Error: unexpected symbol`.

Finally, some functions do not need any arguments to work. A good example is the `Sys.time()` which returns the current time and date. This is useful when using R to generate and update reports automatically. Including this means you can always be clear on when the results were last updated.

```
Sys.time()
```

```
## [1] "2020-09-15 15:13:03 BST"
```

2.3.4 Working with objects

To save an object in our Environment we use the assignment arrow:

```
a <- 103
```

This reads: the object `a` is assigned value 103. `<-` is called "the arrow assignment operator", or "assignment arrow" for short.

Keyboard shortcuts to insert `<-`:
Windows: Alt-
macOS: Option-

You know that the assignment worked when it shows up in the Environment tab. If we now run `a` just on its own, it gets printed back to us:

```
a
```

```
## [1] 103
```

Similarly, if we run a function without assignment to an object, it gets printed but not saved in your Environment:

```
seq(15, 30)
```

```
##  [1] 15 16 17 18 19 20 21 22 23 24 25 26 27 28 29 30
```

`seq()` is a function that creates a sequence of numbers (+1 by default) between the two arguments you pass to it in its brackets. We can assign the result of `seq(15, 30)` into an object, let's call it `example_sequence`:

```
example_sequence <- seq(15, 30)
```

Doing this creates example_sequence in our Environment, but it does not print it. To get it printed, run it on a separate line like this:

```
example_sequence
```

```
##  [1] 15 16 17 18 19 20 21 22 23 24 25 26 27 28 29 30
```

If you save the results of an R function in an object, it does not get printed. If you run a function without the assignment (<-), its results get printed, but not saved as an object.

Finally, R doesn't mind overwriting an existing object, for example:

```
example_sequence <- example_sequence/2
```

```
example_sequence
```

```
##  [1]  7.5  8.0  8.5  9.0  9.5 10.0 10.5 11.0 11.5 12.0 12.5 13.0 13.5 14.0 14.5
## [16] 15.0
```

Notice how we then include the variable on a new line to get it printed as well as overwritten.

2.3.5 <- and =

Note that many people use = instead of <-. Both <- and = can save what is on the right into an object with named on the left. Although <- and = are interchangeable when saving an object into your Environment, they are not interchangeable when used as function argument. For example, remember how we used the na.rm argument in the mean() function, and the result got printed immediately? If we want to save the result into an object, we'll do this, where mean_result could be any name you choose:

```
mean_result <- mean(mydata$var2, na.rm = TRUE)
```

Note how the example above uses both operators: the assignment arrow for saving the result to the Environment, the = equals operator for setting an argument in the mean() function (na.rm = TRUE).

2.3.6   Recap: object, function, input, argument

- To summarise, objects and functions work hand in hand. Objects are both an input as well as the output of a function (what the function returns).

- When passing data to a function, it is usually the first argument, with further arguments used to specify behaviour.

- When we say "the function returns", we are referring to its output (or an Error if it's one of those days).

- The returned object can be different to its input object. In our `mean()` examples above, the input object was a column (`mydata$var1`: 4, 1, 2, 3), whereas the output was a single value: 2.5.

- If you've written a line of code that doesn't include the assignment arrow (`<-`), its results would get printed. If you use the assignment arrow, an object holding the results will get saved into the Environment.

2.4   Pipe - %>%

The pipe - denoted `%>%` - is probably the oddest looking thing you'll see in this book. But please bear with us; it is not as scary as it looks! Furthermore, it is super useful. We use the pipe to send objects into functions.

In the above examples, we calculated the mean of column `var1` from `mydata` by `mean(mydata$var1)`. With the pipe, we can rewrite this as:

```
library(tidyverse)
mydata$var1 %>% mean()
```

```
## [1] 2.5
```

Which reads: "Working with `mydata`, we select a single column called `var1` (with the `$`) **and then** calculate the `mean()`." The pipe becomes especially useful once the analysis includes multiple steps applied one after another. A good way to read and think of the pipe is "and then".

This piping business is not standard R functionality and before using it in a script, you need to tell R this is what you will be doing. The pipe comes from the `magrittr` package (Figure 2.5), but loading the **tidyverse** will also load the pipe. So `library(tidyverse)` initialises everything you need.

To insert a pipe %>%, use the keyboard shortcut ctrl+Shift+M.

With or without the pipe, the general rule "if the result gets printed it doesn't get saved" still applies. To save the result of the function into a new object (so it shows up in the Environment), you need to add the name of the new object with the assignment arrow (<-):

```
mean_result <- mydata$var1 %>% mean()
```

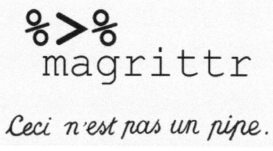

FIGURE 2.5: This is not a pipe. René Magritte inspired artwork, by Stefan Milton Bache.

2.4.1 Using . to direct the pipe

By default, the pipe sends data to the beginning of the function brackets (as most of the functions we use expect data as the first argument). So mydata %>% lm(dependent~explanatory) is equivalent to lm(mydata, dependent~explanatory). lm() - linear model - will be introduced in detail in Chapter 7.

However, the lm() function does not expect data as its first argument. lm() wants us to specify the variables first (dependent~explanatory), and then wants the tibble these columns are in. So we have to use the . to tell the pipe to send the data to the second argument of lm(), not the first, e.g.,

```
mydata %>%
  lm(var1~var2, data = .)
```

2.5 Operators for filtering data

Operators are symbols that tell R how to handle different pieces of data or objects. We have already introduced three: $ (selects a column), <- (assigns values or results to a variable), and the pipe - %>% (sends data into a function).

Other common operators are the ones we use for filtering data - these are arithmetic comparison and logical operators. This may be for creating subgroups, or for excluding outliers or incomplete cases.

The comparison operators that work with numeric data are relatively straightforward: >, <, >=, <=. The first two check whether your values are greater or less than another value, the last two check for "greater than or equal to" and "less than or equal to". These operators are most commonly spotted inside the filter() function:

```
gbd_short %>%
  filter(year < 1995)
```

```
## # A tibble: 3 x 3
##    year cause                    deaths_millions
##    <dbl> <chr>                              <dbl>
## 1  1990 Communicable diseases               15.4
## 2  1990 Injuries                             4.25
## 3  1990 Non-communicable diseases           26.7
```

Here we send the data (gbd_short) to the filter() and ask it to retain all years that are less than 1995. The resulting tibble only includes the year 1990. Now, if we use the <= (less than or equal to) operator, both 1990 and 1995 pass the filter:

```
gbd_short %>%
  filter(year <= 1995)
```

```
## # A tibble: 6 x 3
##    year cause                    deaths_millions
##    <dbl> <chr>                              <dbl>
## 1  1990 Communicable diseases               15.4
## 2  1990 Injuries                             4.25
## 3  1990 Non-communicable diseases           26.7
## 4  1995 Communicable diseases               15.1
## 5  1995 Injuries                             4.53
## 6  1995 Non-communicable diseases           29.3
```

Furthermore, the values either side of the operator could both be variables, e.g., mydata %>% filter(var2 > var1).

To filter for values that are equal to something, we use the == operator.

```
gbd_short %>%
   filter(year == 1995)
```

```
## # A tibble: 3 x 3
##     year cause                        deaths_millions
##    <dbl> <chr>                                  <dbl>
## 1  1995 Communicable diseases                   15.1
## 2  1995 Injuries                                 4.53
## 3  1995 Non-communicable diseases               29.3
```

This reads, take the GBD dataset, send it to the filter and keep rows where year is equal to 1995.

Accidentally using the single equals = when double equals is necessary == is a common mistake and still happens to the best of us. It happens so often that the error the `filter()` function gives when using the wrong one also reminds us what the correct one was:

```
gbd_short %>%
   filter(year = 1995)
```

```
## Error: Problem with `filter()` input `..1`.
## x Input `..1` is named.
## i This usually means that you've used `=` instead of `==`.
## i Did you mean `year == 1995`?
```

The answer to "do you need ==?" is almost always, "Yes R, I do, thank you".

But that's just because `filter()` is a clever cookie and is used to this common mistake. There are other useful functions we use these operators in, but they don't always know to tell us that we've just confused = for ==. So if you get an error when checking for an equality between variables, always check your == operators first.

R also has two operators for combining multiple comparisons: & and |, which stand for AND and OR, respectively. For example, we can filter to only keep the earliest and latest years in the dataset:

```
gbd_short %>%
   filter(year == 1995 | year == 2017)
```

```
## # A tibble: 6 x 3
##     year cause                        deaths_millions
##    <dbl> <chr>                                  <dbl>
## 1  1995 Communicable diseases                   15.1
```

TABLE 2.4: Filtering operators.

Operators	Meaning
==	Equal to
!=	Not equal to
<	Less than
>	Greater than
<=	Less than or equal to
>=	Greater then or equal to
&	AND
|	OR

```
## 2  1995 Injuries                        4.53
## 3  1995 Non-communicable diseases       29.3
## 4  2017 Communicable diseases           10.4
## 5  2017 Injuries                        4.47
## 6  2017 Non-communicable diseases       40.9
```

This reads: take the GBD dataset, send it to the filter and keep rows where year is equal to 1995 OR year is equal to 2017.

Using specific values like we've done here (1995/2017) is called "hard-coding", which is fine if we know for sure that we will not want to use the same script on an updated dataset. But a cleverer way of achieving the same thing is to use the `min()` and `max()` functions:

```
gbd_short %>%
  filter(year == max(year) | year == min(year))
```

```
## # A tibble: 6 x 3
##      year cause                    deaths_millions
##     <dbl> <chr>                              <dbl>
## 1   1990 Communicable diseases              15.4
## 2   1990 Injuries                           4.25
## 3   1990 Non-communicable diseases          26.7
## 4   2017 Communicable diseases              10.4
## 5   2017 Injuries                           4.47
## 6   2017 Non-communicable diseases          40.9
```

2.5.1 Worked examples

Filter the dataset to only include the year 2000. Save this in a new variable using the assignment operator.

```
mydata_year2000 <- gbd_short %>%
  filter(year == 2000)
```

Let's practice combining multiple selections together.

Reminder: '|' means OR and '&' means AND.

From gbd_short, select the lines where year is either 1990 or 2017 and cause is "Communicable diseases":

```
new_data_selection <- gbd_short %>%
  filter((year == 1990 | year == 2013) & cause == "Communicable diseases")

# Or we can get rid of the extra brackets around the years
# by moving cause into a new filter on a new line:

new_data_selection <- gbd_short %>%
  filter(year == 1990 | year == 2013) %>%
  filter(cause == "Communicable diseases")
```

The hash symbol (#) is used to add free text comments to R code. R will not try to run these lines, they will be ignored. Comments are an essential part of any programming code and these are "Dear Diary" notes to your future self.

2.6   The combine function: c()

The combine function as its name implies is used to combine several values. It is especially useful when used with the %in% operator to filter for multiple values. Remember how the gbd_short cause column had three different causes in it:

```
gbd_short$cause %>% unique()
```

```
## [1] "Communicable diseases"     "Injuries"
## [3] "Non-communicable diseases"
```

Say we wanted to filter for communicable and non-communicable diseases. [6] We could use the OR operator | like this:

```
gbd_short %>%
  # also filtering for a single year to keep the result concise
  filter(year == 1990) %>%
  filter(cause == "Communicable diseases" | cause == "Non-communicable diseases")
```

```
## # A tibble: 2 x 3
##    year cause                     deaths_millions
##   <dbl> <chr>                              <dbl>
## 1  1990 Communicable diseases               15.4
## 2  1990 Non-communicable diseases           26.7
```

---

[6]In this example, it would just be easier to used the "not equal" operator, filter(cause != "Injuries"), but imagine your column had more than just three different values in it.

But that means we have to type in `cause` twice (and more if we had other values we wanted to include). This is where the `%in%` operator together with the `c()` function come in handy:

```
gbd_short %>%
  filter(year == 1990) %>%
  filter(cause %in% c("Communicable diseases", "Non-communicable diseases"))
```

```
## # A tibble: 2 x 3
##    year cause                        deaths_millions
##    <dbl> <chr>                                  <dbl>
## 1  1990 Communicable diseases                   15.4
## 2  1990 Non-communicable diseases               26.7
```

2.7 Missing values (NAs) and filters

Filtering for missing values (NAs) needs special attention and care. Remember the small example tibble from Table 2.3 - it has some NAs in columns `var2` and `var3`:

```
mydata
```

```
## # A tibble: 4 x 5
##       id sex       var1  var2  var3
##    <int> <chr>    <dbl> <dbl> <dbl>
## 1     1 Male         4    NA     2
## 2     2 Female       1     4     1
## 3     3 Female       2     5    NA
## 4     4 Male         3    NA    NA
```

If we now want to filter for rows where `var2` is missing, `filter(var2 == NA)` is not the way to do it, it will not work.

Since R is a programming language, it can be a bit stubborn with things like these. When you ask R to do a comparison using `==` (or `<`, `>`, etc.) it expects a value on each side, but NA is not a value, it is the lack thereof. The way to filter for missing values is using the `is.na()` function:

```
mydata %>%
  filter(is.na(var2))
```

```
## # A tibble: 2 x 5
##       id sex       var1  var2  var3
##    <int> <chr>    <dbl> <dbl> <dbl>
## 1     1 Male         4    NA     2
## 2     4 Male         3    NA    NA
```

We send `mydata` to the filter and keep rows where `var2` is NA. Note the double brackets at the end: that's because the inner one belongs to `is.na()`, and the outer one to `filter()`. Missing out a closing bracket is also a common source of errors, and still happens to the best of us.

If filtering for rows where `var2` is not missing, we do this[7]

```
mydata %>%
    filter(!is.na(var2))
```

```
## # A tibble: 2 x 5
##      id sex      var1  var2  var3
##   <int> <chr>  <dbl> <dbl> <dbl>
## 1     2 Female     1     4     1
## 2     3 Female     2     5    NA
```

In R, the exclamation mark (!) means "not".

Sometimes you want to drop a specific value (e.g., an outlier) from the dataset like this. The small example tibble `mydata` has 4 rows, with the values for `var2` as follows: NA, 4, 5, NA. We can exclude the row where `var2` is equal to 5 by using the "not equals" (`!=`)[8]:

```
mydata %>%
    filter(var2 != 5)
```

```
## # A tibble: 1 x 5
##      id sex      var1  var2  var3
##   <int> <chr>  <dbl> <dbl> <dbl>
## 1     2 Female     1     4     1
```

However, you'll see that by doing this, R drops the rows where `var2` is NA as well, as it can't be sure these missing values were not equal to 5.

If you want to keep the missing values, you need to make use of the OR (|) operator and the `is.na()` function:

```
mydata %>%
    filter(var2 != 5 | is.na(var2))
```

```
## # A tibble: 3 x 5
##      id sex      var1  var2  var3
##   <int> <chr>  <dbl> <dbl> <dbl>
## 1     1 Male       4    NA     2
## 2     2 Female     1     4     1
## 3     4 Male       3    NA    NA
```

---

[7]In this simple example, `mydata %>% filter(! is.na(var2))` could be replaced by a shorthand: `mydata %>% drop_na(var2)`, but it is important to understand how the ! and `is.na()` work as there will be more complex situations where using these is necessary.

[8]`filter(var2 != 5)` is equivalent to `filter(! var2 == 5)`

Being caught out by missing values, either in filters or other functions is common (remember `mydata$var2 %>% mean()` returns NA unless you add `na.rm = TRUE`). This is also why we insist that you always plot your data first - outliers will reveal themselves and NA values usually become obvious too.

Another thing we do to stay safe around filters and missing values is saving the results and making sure the number of rows still add up:

```
subset1 <- mydata %>%
  filter(var2 == 5)

subset2 <- mydata %>%
  filter(! var2 == 5)

subset1
```

```
## # A tibble: 1 x 5
##       id sex     var1  var2  var3
##    <int> <chr>  <dbl> <dbl> <dbl>
## 1     3 Female    2     5    NA
```

```
subset2
```

```
## # A tibble: 1 x 5
##       id sex     var1  var2  var3
##    <int> <chr>  <dbl> <dbl> <dbl>
## 1     2 Female    1     4     1
```

If the numbers are small, you can now quickly look at RStudio's Environment tab and figure out whether the number of observations (rows) in `subset1` and `subset2` add up to the whole dataset (`mydata`). Or use the `nrow()` function to check the number of rows in each dataset:

Rows in `mydata`:

```
nrow(mydata)
```

```
## [1] 4
```

Rows in `subset1`:

```
nrow(subset1)
```

```
## [1] 1
```

Rows in `subset2`:

```
nrow(subset2)
```

```
## [1] 1
```

Asking R whether adding these two up equals the original size:

```
nrow(subset1) + nrow(subset2) == nrow(mydata)
```

```
## [1] FALSE
```

As expected, this returns FALSE - because we didn't add special handling for missing values. Let's create a third subset only including rows where var3 is NA:

Rows in subset2:

```
subset3 <- mydata %>%
  filter(is.na(var2))

nrow(subset1) + nrow(subset2) + nrow(subset3) == nrow(mydata)
```

```
## [1] TRUE
```

2.8   Creating new columns - mutate()

The function for adding new columns (or making changes to existing ones) to a tibble is called mutate(). As a reminder, this is what typesdata looked like:

```
typesdata
```

```
## # A tibble: 3 x 4
##    id    group      measurement date
##    <chr> <chr>            <dbl> <dttm>
## 1 ID1    Control            1.8 2017-01-02 12:00:00
## 2 ID2    Treatment          4.5 2018-02-03 13:00:00
## 3 ID3    Treatment          3.7 2019-03-04 14:00:00
```

Let's say we decide to divide the column measurement by 2. A quick way to see these values would be to pull them out using the $ operator and then divide by 2:

```
typesdata$measurement
```

```
## [1] 1.8 4.5 3.7
```

```
typesdata$measurement/2
```

```
## [1] 0.90 2.25 1.85
```

But this becomes cumbersome once we want to combine multiple variables from the same tibble in a calculation. So the `mutate()` is the way to go here:

```
typesdata %>%
  mutate(measurement/2)
```

```
## # A tibble: 3 x 5
##    id    group    measurement date                `measurement/2`
##    <chr> <chr>          <dbl> <dttm>                         <dbl>
## 1 ID1   Control          1.8 2017-01-02 12:00:00            0.9
## 2 ID2   Treatment        4.5 2018-02-03 13:00:00            2.25
## 3 ID3   Treatment        3.7 2019-03-04 14:00:00            1.85
```

Notice how the `mutate()` above returns the whole tibble with a new column called `measurement/2`. This is quite nice of `mutate()`, but it would be best to give columns names that don't include characters other than underscores (_) or dots (.). So let's assign a more standard name for this new column:

```
typesdata %>%
  mutate(measurement_half = measurement/2)
```

```
## # A tibble: 3 x 5
##    id    group    measurement date                measurement_half
##    <chr> <chr>          <dbl> <dttm>                          <dbl>
## 1 ID1   Control          1.8 2017-01-02 12:00:00             0.9
## 2 ID2   Treatment        4.5 2018-02-03 13:00:00             2.25
## 3 ID3   Treatment        3.7 2019-03-04 14:00:00             1.85
```

Better. You can see that R likes the name we gave it a bit better as it's now removed the back-ticks from around it. Overall, back-ticks can be used to call out non-standard column names, so if you are forced to read in data with, e.g., spaces in column names, then the back-ticks enable calling column names that would otherwise error[9]:

```
mydata$`Nasty column name`
```

```
# or
```

```
mydata %>%
  select(`Nasty column name`)
```

But as usual, if it gets printed, it doesn't get saved. We have two options - we

---

[9]If this happens to you a lot, then check out `library(janitor)` and its function `clean_names()` for automatically tidying non-standard column names.

can either overwrite the `typesdata` tibble (by changing the first line to `typesdata =`
`typesdata %>%`), or we can create a new one (that appears in your Environment):

```
typesdata_modified <- typesdata %>%
  mutate(measurement_half = measurement/2)

typesdata_modified
```

```
## # A tibble: 3 x 5
##   id    group    measurement date                measurement_half
##   <chr> <chr>          <dbl> <dttm>                         <dbl>
## 1 ID1   Control          1.8 2017-01-02 12:00:00             0.9
## 2 ID2   Treatment        4.5 2018-02-03 13:00:00             2.25
## 3 ID3   Treatment        3.7 2019-03-04 14:00:00             1.85
```

The `mutate()` function can also be used to create a new column with a single
constant value; which in return can be used to calculate a difference for each
of the existing dates:

```
library(lubridate)
typesdata %>%
  mutate(reference_date   = ymd_hm("2020-01-01 12:00"),
         dates_difference = reference_date - date) %>%
  select(date, reference_date, dates_difference)
```

```
## # A tibble: 3 x 3
##   date                reference_date      dates_difference
##   <dttm>              <dttm>              <drtn>
## 1 2017-01-02 12:00:00 2020-01-01 12:00:00 1094.0000 days
## 2 2018-02-03 13:00:00 2020-01-01 12:00:00  696.9583 days
## 3 2019-03-04 14:00:00 2020-01-01 12:00:00  302.9167 days
```

(We are then using the `select()` function to only choose the three relevant
columns.)

Finally, the mutate function can be used to create a new column with a summarised value in it, e.g., the mean of another column:

```
typesdata %>%
  mutate(mean_measurement = mean(measurement))
```

```
## # A tibble: 3 x 5
##   id    group    measurement date                mean_measurement
##   <chr> <chr>          <dbl> <dttm>                         <dbl>
## 1 ID1   Control          1.8 2017-01-02 12:00:00            3.33
## 2 ID2   Treatment        4.5 2018-02-03 13:00:00            3.33
## 3 ID3   Treatment        3.7 2019-03-04 14:00:00            3.33
```

Which in return can be useful for calculating a standardized measurement (i.e.,
relative to the mean):

```
typesdata %>%
  mutate(mean_measurement     = mean(measurement)) %>%
  mutate(measurement_relative = measurement/mean_measurement) %>%
  select(matches("measurement"))
```

```
## # A tibble: 3 x 3
##    measurement mean_measurement measurement_relative
##          <dbl>            <dbl>                <dbl>
## 1          1.8             3.33                 0.54
## 2          4.5             3.33                 1.35
## 3          3.7             3.33                 1.11
```

2.8.1   Worked example/exercise

Round the difference to 0 decimal places using the `round()` function inside a `mutate()`. Then add a clever `matches("date")` inside the `select()` function to choose all matching columns.

Solution:

```
typesdata %>%
  mutate(reference_date   = ymd_hm("2020-01-01 12:00"),
         dates_difference = reference_date - date) %>%
  mutate(dates_difference = round(dates_difference)) %>%
  select(matches("date"))
```

```
## # A tibble: 3 x 3
##    date                reference_date      dates_difference
##    <dttm>              <dttm>              <drtn>
## 1 2017-01-02 12:00:00 2020-01-01 12:00:00 1094 days
## 2 2018-02-03 13:00:00 2020-01-01 12:00:00  697 days
## 3 2019-03-04 14:00:00 2020-01-01 12:00:00  303 days
```

You can shorten this by adding the `round()` function directly around the subtraction, so the third line becomes `dates_difference = round(reference_date - date)` `%>%`. But sometimes writing calculations out longer than the absolute minimum can make them easier to understand when you return to an old script months later.

Furthermore, we didn't have to save the `reference_date` as a new column, the calculation could have used the value directly: `mutate(dates_difference = ymd_hm("2020-01-01 12:00") - date) %>%`. But again, defining it makes it clearer for your future self to see what was done. And it makes `reference_date` available for reuse in more complicated calculations within the tibble.

2.9 Conditional calculations - `if_else()`

And finally, we combine the filtering operators (`==`, `>`, `<`, etc) with the `if_else()` function to create new columns based on a condition.

```
typesdata %>%
  mutate(above_threshold = if_else(measurement > 3,
                                   "Above three",
                                   "Below three"))
```

```
## # A tibble: 3 x 5
##   id    group     measurement date                above_threshold
##   <chr> <chr>           <dbl> <dttm>              <chr>
## 1 ID1   Control           1.8 2017-01-02 12:00:00 Below three
## 2 ID2   Treatment         4.5 2018-02-03 13:00:00 Above three
## 3 ID3   Treatment         3.7 2019-03-04 14:00:00 Above three
```

We are sending `typesdata` into a `mutate()` function, we are creating a new column called `above_threshold` based on whether `measurement` is greater or less than 3. The first argument to `if_else()` is a condition (in this case that measurement is greater than 3), the second argument is the value if the condition is TRUE, and the third argument is the value if the condition is FALSE.

It reads, "if this condition is met, return this, else return that".

Look at each line in the tibble above and convince yourself that the `threshold` variable worked as expected. Then look at the two closing brackets - `))` - at the end and convince yourself that they are both needed.

`if_else()` and missing values tip: for rows with missing values (NAs), the condition returns neither TRUE nor FALSE, it returns NA. And that might be fine, but if you want to assign a specific group/label for missing values in the new variable, you can add a fourth argument to `if_else()`, e.g., `if_else(measurement > 3, "Above three", "Below three", "Value missing")`.

2.10 Create labels - `paste()`

The `paste()` function is used to add characters together. It also works with numbers and dates which will automatically be converted to characters before being pasted together into a single label. See this example where we use all

variables from `typesdata` to create a new column called `plot_label` (we `select()`
for printing space):

```
typesdata %>%
  mutate(plot_label = paste(id,
                            "was last measured at", date,
                            ", and the value was",    measurement)) %>%
  select(plot_label)
```

```
## # A tibble: 3 x 1
##   plot_label
##   <chr>
## 1 ID1 was last measured at 2017-01-02 12:00:00 , and the value was 1.8
## 2 ID2 was last measured at 2018-02-03 13:00:00 , and the value was 4.5
## 3 ID3 was last measured at 2019-03-04 14:00:00 , and the value was 3.7
```

The paste is also useful when pieces of information are stored in different
columns. For example, consider this made-up tibble:

```
pastedata <- tibble(year  = c(2007, 2008, 2009),
                    month = c("Jan", "Feb", "March"),
                    day   = c(1, 2, 3))

pastedata
```

```
## # A tibble: 3 x 3
##    year month   day
##   <dbl> <chr> <dbl>
## 1  2007 Jan       1
## 2  2008 Feb       2
## 3  2009 March     3
```

We can use `paste()` to combine these into a single column:

```
pastedata %>%
  mutate(date = paste(day, month, year, sep = "-"))
```

```
## # A tibble: 3 x 4
##    year month   day date
##   <dbl> <chr> <dbl> <chr>
## 1  2007 Jan       1 1-Jan-2007
## 2  2008 Feb       2 2-Feb-2008
## 3  2009 March     3 3-March-2009
```

By default, `paste()` adds a space between each value, but we can use the `sep =`
argument to specify a different separator. Sometimes it is useful to use `paste0()`
which does not add anything between the values (no space, no dash, etc.).

We can now tell R that the date column should be parsed as such:

```
library(lubridate)

pastedata %>%
  mutate(date = paste(day, month, year, sep = "-")) %>%
  mutate(date = dmy(date))
```

```
## # A tibble: 3 x 4
##    year month   day date
##   <dbl> <chr> <dbl> <date>
## 1  2007 Jan       1 2007-01-01
## 2  2008 Feb       2 2008-02-02
## 3  2009 March     3 2009-03-03
```

2.11   Joining multiple datasets

It is common for different pieces of information to be kept in different files or
tables and you often want to combine them together. For example, consider
you have some demographic information (id, sex, age) in one file:

```
library(tidyverse)
patientdata <- read_csv("data/patient_data.csv")
patientdata
```

```
## # A tibble: 6 x 3
##       id sex       age
##    <dbl> <chr>   <dbl>
## 1      1 Female     24
## 2      2 Male       59
## 3      3 Female     32
## 4      4 Female     84
## 5      5 Male       48
## 6      6 Female     65
```

And another one with some lab results (id, measurement):

```
labsdata <- read_csv("data/labs_data.csv")
labsdata
```

```
## # A tibble: 4 x 2
##       id measurement
##    <dbl>       <dbl>
## 1      5        3.47
## 2      6        7.31
## 3      8        9.91
## 4      7        6.11
```

Notice how these datasets are not only different sizes (6 rows in patientdata, 4 rows in `labsdata`), but include information on different patients: `patiendata` has ids 1, 2, 3, 4, 5, 6, `labsdata` has ids 5, 6, 8, 7.

A comprehensive way to join these is to use `full_join()` retaining all information from both tibbles (and matching up rows by shared columns, in this case `id`):

```
full_join(patientdata, labsdata)
```

```
## Joining, by = "id"
## # A tibble: 8 x 4
##       id sex       age measurement
##    <dbl> <chr>   <dbl>       <dbl>
## 1      1 Female     24          NA
## 2      2 Male       59          NA
## 3      3 Female     32          NA
## 4      4 Female     84          NA
## 5      5 Male       48        3.47
## 6      6 Female     65        7.31
## 7      8 <NA>       NA        9.91
## 8      7 <NA>       NA        6.11
```

However, if we are only interested in matching information, we use the inner join:

```
inner_join(patientdata, labsdata)
```

```
## Joining, by = "id"
## # A tibble: 2 x 4
##       id sex       age measurement
##    <dbl> <chr>   <dbl>       <dbl>
## 1      5 Male       48        3.47
## 2      6 Female     65        7.31
```

And finally, if we want to retain all information from one tibble, we use either the `left_join()` or the `right_join()`:

```
left_join(patientdata, labsdata)
```

```
## Joining, by = "id"
## # A tibble: 6 x 4
##       id sex       age measurement
##    <dbl> <chr>   <dbl>       <dbl>
## 1      1 Female     24          NA
## 2      2 Male       59          NA
## 3      3 Female     32          NA
## 4      4 Female     84          NA
## 5      5 Male       48        3.47
## 6      6 Female     65        7.31
```

```
right_join(patientdata, labsdata)
```

```
## Joining, by = "id"
```

```
## # A tibble: 4 x 4
##      id sex       age measurement
##   <dbl> <chr>   <dbl>       <dbl>
## 1     5 Male       48        3.47
## 2     6 Female     65        7.31
## 3     8 <NA>       NA        9.91
## 4     7 <NA>       NA        6.11
```

2.11.1 Further notes about joins

- The joins functions (`full_join()`, `inner_join()`, `left_join()`, `right_join()`) will automatically look for matching column names. You can use the `by =` argument
to specify by hand. This is especially useful if the columns are named differently in the datasets, e.g., `left_join(data1, data2, by = c("id" = "patient_id"))`.

- The rows do not have to be ordered, the joins match on values within the
rows, not the order of the rows within the tibble.

- Joins are used to combine different variables (columns) into a single tibble.
If you are getting more data of the same variables, use `bind_rows()`
instead:

```
patientdata_new <- read_csv("data/patient_data_updated.csv")
patientdata_new
```

```
## # A tibble: 2 x 3
##      id sex       age
##   <dbl> <chr>   <dbl>
## 1     7 Female     38
## 2     8 Male       29
```

```
bind_rows(patientdata, patientdata_new)
```

```
## # A tibble: 8 x 3
##      id sex       age
##   <dbl> <chr>   <dbl>
## 1     1 Female     24
## 2     2 Male       59
## 3     3 Female     32
## 4     4 Female     84
## 5     5 Male       48
## 6     6 Female     65
## 7     7 Female     38
## 8     8 Male       29
```

Finally, it is important to understand how joins behave if there are multiple matches within the tibbles. For example, if patient id 4 had a second measurement as well:

```
labsdata_updated <- labsdata %>%
   add_row(id = 5, measurement = 2.49)
labsdata_updated
```

```
## # A tibble: 5 x 2
##       id measurement
##    <dbl>       <dbl>
## 1      5        3.47
## 2      6        7.31
## 3      8        9.91
## 4      7        6.11
## 5      5        2.49
```

When we now do a left_join() with our main tibble - patientdata:

```
left_join(patientdata, labsdata_updated)
```

```
## Joining, by = "id"
## # A tibble: 7 x 4
##       id sex      age measurement
##    <dbl> <chr>  <dbl>       <dbl>
## 1      1 Female    24          NA
## 2      2 Male      59          NA
## 3      3 Female    32          NA
## 4      4 Female    84          NA
## 5      5 Male      48        3.47
## 6      5 Male      48        2.49
## 7      6 Female    65        7.31
```

We get 7 rows, instead of 6 - as patient id 5 now appears twice with the two different measurements. So it is important to either know your datasets well or keep an eye on the number of rows to make sure any increases/decreases in the tibble sizes are as you expect them to be.

3

Summarising data

"The Answer to the Great Question ... Of Life, the Universe and Everything
... Is ... Forty-two," said Deep Thought, with infinite majesty and calm.
Douglas Adams, The Hitchhiker's Guide to the Galaxy

In this chapter you will find out how to:

- summarise data using: `group_by()`, `summarise()`, and `mutate()`;
- reshape data between the wide and long formats: `pivot_wider()` and `pivot_longer()`;
- `select()` columns and `arrange()` (sort) rows.

The exercises at the end of this chapter combine all of the above to give context and show you more worked examples.

3.1 Get the data

Dataset: Global Burden of Disease (year, cause, sex, income, deaths)

The Global Burden of Disease dataset used in this chapter is more detailed than the one we used previously. For each year, the total number of deaths from the three broad disease categories are also separated into sex and World Bank income categories. This means that we have 24 rows for each year, and that the total number of deaths per year is the sum of these 24 rows:

```
library(tidyverse)
gbd_full <- read_csv("data/global_burden_disease_cause-year-sex-income.csv")

# Creating a single-year tibble for printing and simple examples:
gbd2017 <- gbd_full %>%
  filter(year == 2017)
```

TABLE 3.1: Deaths per year (2017) from three broad disease categories, sex, and World Bank country-level income groups.

cause	year	sex	income	deaths_millions
Communicable diseases	2017	Female	High	0.26
Communicable diseases	2017	Female	Upper-Middle	0.55
Communicable diseases	2017	Female	Lower-Middle	2.92
Communicable diseases	2017	Female	Low	1.18
Communicable diseases	2017	Male	High	0.29
Communicable diseases	2017	Male	Upper-Middle	0.73
Communicable diseases	2017	Male	Lower-Middle	3.10
Communicable diseases	2017	Male	Low	1.35
Injuries	2017	Female	High	0.21
Injuries	2017	Female	Upper-Middle	0.43
Injuries	2017	Female	Lower-Middle	0.66
Injuries	2017	Female	Low	0.12
Injuries	2017	Male	High	0.40
Injuries	2017	Male	Upper-Middle	1.16
Injuries	2017	Male	Lower-Middle	1.23
Injuries	2017	Male	Low	0.26
Non-communicable diseases	2017	Female	High	4.68
Non-communicable diseases	2017	Female	Upper-Middle	7.28
Non-communicable diseases	2017	Female	Lower-Middle	6.27
Non-communicable diseases	2017	Female	Low	0.92
Non-communicable diseases	2017	Male	High	4.65
Non-communicable diseases	2017	Male	Upper-Middle	8.79
Non-communicable diseases	2017	Male	Lower-Middle	7.30
Non-communicable diseases	2017	Male	Low	1.00

3.2 Plot the data

The best way to investigate a dataset is of course to plot it. We have added a couple of notes as comments (the lines starting with a #) for those who can't wait to get to the next chapter where the code for plotting will be introduced and explained in detail. Overall, you shouldn't waste time trying to understand this code, but do look at the different groups within this new dataset.

```
gbd2017 %>%
  # without the mutate(... = fct_relevel())
  # the panels get ordered alphabetically
  mutate(income = fct_relevel(income,
                     "Low",
                     "Lower-Middle",
                     "Upper-Middle",
                     "High")) %>%
  # defining the variables using ggplot(aes(...)):
  ggplot(aes(x = sex, y = deaths_millions, fill = cause)) +
  # type of geom to be used: column (that's a type of barplot):
  geom_col(position = "dodge") +
  # facets for the income groups:
  facet_wrap(~income, ncol = 4) +
  # move the legend to the top of the plot (default is "right"):
  theme(legend.position = "top")
```

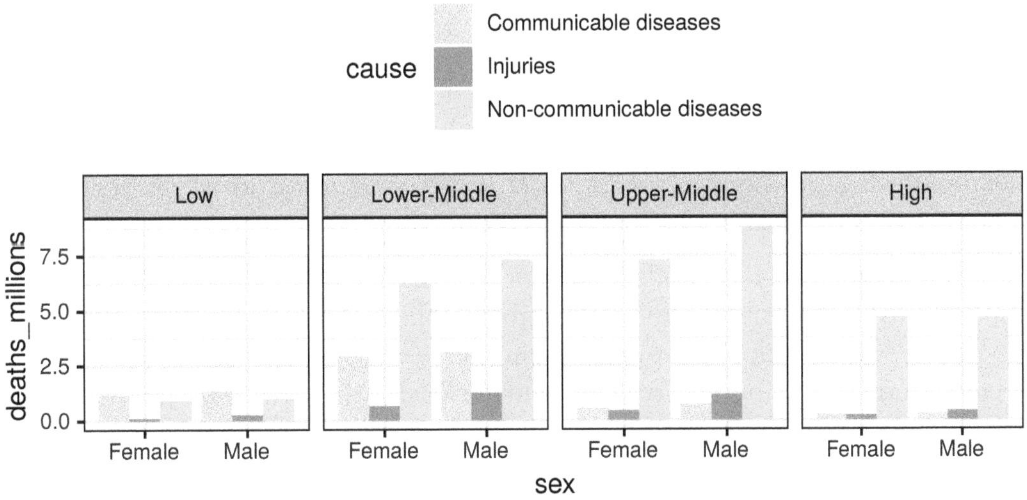

FIGURE 3.1: Global Burden of Disease data with subgroups: cause, sex, World Bank income group.

3.3 Aggregating: `group_by()`, `summarise()`

Health data analysis is frequently concerned with making comparisons between groups. Groups of genes, or diseases, or patients, or populations, etc. An easy approach to the comparison of data by a categorical grouping is therefore essential.

We will introduce flexible functions from **tidyverse** that you can apply in any setting. The examples intentionally get quite involved to demonstrate the different approaches that can be used.

To quickly calculate the total number of deaths in 2017, we can select the column and send it into the `sum()` function:

```
gbd2017$deaths_millions %>% sum()
```

```
## [1] 55.74
```

But a much cleverer way of summarising data is using the `summarise()` function:

```
gbd2017 %>%
  summarise(sum(deaths_millions))
```

```
## # A tibble: 1 x 1
##    `sum(deaths_millions)`
##                     <dbl>
## 1                   55.74
```

This is indeed equal to the number of deaths per year we saw in the previous chapter using the shorter version of this data (deaths from the three causes were 10.38, 4.47, 40.89 which adds to 55.74).

`sum()` is a function that adds numbers together, whereas `summarise()` is an efficient way of creating summarised tibbles. The main strength of `summarise()` is how it works with the `group_by()` function. `group_by()` and `summarise()` are like cheese and wine, a perfect complement for each other, seldom seen apart.

We use `group_by()` to tell `summarise()` which subgroups to apply the calculations on. In the above example, without `group_by()`, summarise just works on the whole dataset, yielding the same result as just sending a single column into the `sum()` function.

We can subset on the cause variable using `group_by()`:

```
gbd2017 %>%
  group_by(cause) %>%
  summarise(sum(deaths_millions))
```

```
## `summarise()` ungrouping output (override with `.groups` argument)

## # A tibble: 3 x 2
##   cause                    `sum(deaths_millions)`
##   <chr>                                     <dbl>
## 1 Communicable diseases                     10.38
## 2 Injuries                                   4.47
## 3 Non-communicable diseases                 40.89
```

Furthermore, `group_by()` is happy to accept multiple grouping variables. So by just copying and editing the above code, we can quickly get summarised totals across multiple grouping variables (by just adding `sex` inside the `group_by()` after `cause`):

```
gbd2017 %>%
  group_by(cause, sex) %>%
  summarise(sum(deaths_millions))
```

```
## `summarise()` regrouping output by 'cause' (override with `.groups` argument)

## # A tibble: 6 x 3
## # Groups:   cause [3]
##   cause                     sex     `sum(deaths_millions)`
##   <chr>                     <chr>                    <dbl>
## 1 Communicable diseases     Female                    4.91
## 2 Communicable diseases     Male                      5.47
## 3 Injuries                  Female                    1.42
## 4 Injuries                  Male                      3.05
## 5 Non-communicable diseases Female                   19.15
## 6 Non-communicable diseases Male                     21.74
```

3.4 Add new columns: `mutate()`

We met `mutate()` in the last chapter. Let's first give the summarised column a better name, e.g., `deaths_per_group`. We can remove groupings by using `ungroup()`. This is important to remember if you want to manipulate the dataset in its original format. We can combine `ungroup()` with `mutate()` to add a total deaths column, which will be used below to calculate a percentage:

```
gbd2017 %>%
  group_by(cause, sex) %>%
  summarise(deaths_per_group = sum(deaths_millions)) %>%
```

```
ungroup() %>%
mutate(deaths_total = sum(deaths_per_group))
```

```
## `summarise()` regrouping output by 'cause' (override with `.groups` argument)
## # A tibble: 6 x 4
##   cause                    sex    deaths_per_group deaths_total
##   <chr>                    <chr>             <dbl>        <dbl>
## 1 Communicable diseases    Female             4.91        55.74
## 2 Communicable diseases    Male               5.47        55.74
## 3 Injuries                 Female             1.42        55.74
## 4 Injuries                 Male               3.05        55.74
## 5 Non-communicable diseases Female           19.15        55.74
## 6 Non-communicable diseases Male             21.74        55.74
```

3.4.1 Percentages formatting: `percent()`

So `summarise()` condenses a tibble, whereas `mutate()` retains its current size and adds columns. We can also further lines to `mutate()` to calculate the percentage of each group:

```
# percent() function for formatting percentages come from library(scales)
library(scales)
gbd2017_summarised <- gbd2017 %>%
  group_by(cause, sex) %>%
  summarise(deaths_per_group = sum(deaths_millions)) %>%
  ungroup() %>%
  mutate(deaths_total    = sum(deaths_per_group),
         deaths_relative = percent(deaths_per_group/deaths_total))
gbd2017_summarised
```

```
## # A tibble: 6 x 5
##   cause                    sex    deaths_per_group deaths_total deaths_relative
##   <chr>                    <chr>             <dbl>        <dbl> <chr>
## 1 Communicable diseases    Female             4.91        55.74 8.8%
## 2 Communicable diseases    Male               5.47        55.74 9.8%
## 3 Injuries                 Female             1.42        55.74 2.5%
## 4 Injuries                 Male               3.05        55.74 5.5%
## 5 Non-communicable diseases Female           19.15        55.74 34.4%
## 6 Non-communicable diseases Male             21.74        55.74 39.0%
```

The `percent()` function comes from `library(scales)` and is a handy way of formatting percentages You must keep in mind that it changes the column from a number (denoted `<dbl>`) to a character (`<chr>`). The `percent()` function is equivalent to:

```
# using values from the first row as an example:
round(100*4.91/55.74, 1) %>% paste0("%")
```

```
## [1] "8.8%"
```

This is convenient for final presentation of number, but if you intend to do further calculations/plot/sort the percentages just calculate them as fractions with:

```
gbd2017_summarised %>%
  mutate(deaths_relative = deaths_per_group/deaths_total)
```

```
## # A tibble: 6 x 5
##   cause                      sex    deaths_per_group deaths_total deaths_relative
##   <chr>                      <chr>             <dbl>        <dbl>           <dbl>
## 1 Communicable diseases      Female             4.91        55.74         0.08809
## 2 Communicable diseases      Male               5.47        55.74         0.09813
## 3 Injuries                   Female             1.42        55.74         0.02548
## 4 Injuries                   Male               3.05        55.74         0.05472
## 5 Non-communicable diseases Female            19.15        55.74         0.3436
## 6 Non-communicable diseases Male              21.74        55.74         0.3900
```

and convert to nicely formatted percentages later with `mutate(deaths_percentage = percent(deaths_relative))`.

3.5 `summarise()` vs `mutate()`

So far we've shown you examples of using `summarise()` on grouped data (following `group_by()`) and `mutate()` on the whole dataset (without using `group_by()`).

But here's the thing: `mutate()` is also happy to work on grouped data.

Let's save the aggregated example from above in a new tibble. We will then sort the rows using `arrange()` based on `sex`, just for easier viewing (it was previously sorted by `cause`).

The `arrange()` function sorts the rows within a tibble:

```
gbd_summarised <- gbd2017 %>%
  group_by(cause, sex) %>%
  summarise(deaths_per_group = sum(deaths_millions)) %>%
  arrange(sex)
```

```
## `summarise()` regrouping output by 'cause' (override with `.groups` argument)
```

```
gbd_summarised
```

```
## # A tibble: 6 x 3
## # Groups:   cause [3]
##   cause                      sex    deaths_per_group
##   <chr>                      <chr>             <dbl>
## 1 Communicable diseases      Female             4.91
```

```
## 2 Injuries                    Female          1.42
## 3 Non-communicable diseases Female         19.15
## 4 Communicable diseases      Male           5.47
## 5 Injuries                   Male           3.05
## 6 Non-communicable diseases Male           21.74
```

You should also notice that `summarise()` drops all variables that are not listed in `group_by()` or created inside it. So `year`, `income`, and `deaths_millions` exist in `gbd2017`, but they do not exist in `gbd_summarised`.

We now want to calculate the percentage of deaths from each cause for each gender. We could use `summarise()` to calculate the totals:

```
gbd_summarised_sex <- gbd_summarised %>%
  group_by(sex) %>%
  summarise(deaths_per_sex = sum(deaths_per_group))
```

```
## `summarise()` ungrouping output (override with `.groups` argument)
```

```
gbd_summarised_sex
```

```
## # A tibble: 2 x 2
##   sex     deaths_per_sex
##   <chr>          <dbl>
## 1 Female         25.48
## 2 Male           30.26
```

But that drops the `cause` and `deaths_per_group` columns. One way would be to now use a join on `gbd_summarised` and `gbd_summarised_sex`:

```
full_join(gbd_summarised, gbd_summarised_sex)
```

```
## Joining, by = "sex"
```

```
## # A tibble: 6 x 4
## # Groups:   cause [3]
##   cause                    sex     deaths_per_group deaths_per_sex
##   <chr>                    <chr>          <dbl>          <dbl>
## 1 Communicable diseases    Female          4.91          25.48
## 2 Injuries                 Female          1.42          25.48
## 3 Non-communicable diseases Female        19.15          25.48
## 4 Communicable diseases    Male            5.47          30.26
## 5 Injuries                 Male            3.05          30.26
## 6 Non-communicable diseases Male          21.74          30.26
```

Joining different summaries together can be useful, especially if the individual pipelines are quite long (e.g., over 5 lines of `%>%`). However, it does increase the chance of mistakes creeping in and is best avoided if possible.

An alternative is to use `mutate()` with `group_by()` to achieve the same result as the `full_join()` above:

```
gbd_summarised %>%
  group_by(sex) %>%
  mutate(deaths_per_sex = sum(deaths_per_group))
```

```
## # A tibble: 6 x 4
## # Groups:   sex [2]
##    cause                      sex    deaths_per_group deaths_per_sex
##    <chr>                      <chr>             <dbl>          <dbl>
## 1 Communicable diseases       Female             4.91          25.48
## 2 Injuries                    Female             1.42          25.48
## 3 Non-communicable diseases Female              19.15          25.48
## 4 Communicable diseases       Male               5.47          30.26
## 5 Injuries                    Male               3.05          30.26
## 6 Non-communicable diseases Male               21.74          30.26
```

So `mutate()` calculates the sums within each grouping variable (in this example just `group_by(sex)`) and puts the results in a new column without condensing the tibble down or removing any of the existing columns.

Let's combine all of this together into a single pipeline and calculate the percentages per cause for each gender:

```
gbd2017 %>%
  group_by(cause, sex) %>%
  summarise(deaths_per_group = sum(deaths_millions)) %>%
  group_by(sex) %>%
  mutate(deaths_per_sex  = sum(deaths_per_group),
         sex_cause_perc = percent(deaths_per_group/deaths_per_sex)) %>%
  arrange(sex, deaths_per_group)
```

```
## `summarise()` regrouping output by 'cause' (override with `.groups` argument)
```

```
## # A tibble: 6 x 5
## # Groups:   sex [2]
##    cause                      sex    deaths_per_group deaths_per_sex sex_cause_perc
##    <chr>                      <chr>             <dbl>          <dbl> <chr>
## 1 Injuries                    Fema~              1.42          25.48 6%
## 2 Communicable diseases       Fema~              4.91          25.48 19%
## 3 Non-communicable diseases Fema~              19.15          25.48 75%
## 4 Injuries                    Male               3.05          30.26 10.1%
## 5 Communicable diseases       Male               5.47          30.26 18.1%
## 6 Non-communicable diseases Male               21.74          30.26 71.8%
```

3.6 Common arithmetic functions - `sum()`, `mean()`, `median()`, etc.

Statistics is an R strength, so if there is an arithmetic function you can think of, it probably exists in R.

The most common ones are:

- `sum()`
- `mean()`
- `median()`
- `min()`, `max()`
- `sd()` - standard deviation
- `IQR()` - interquartile range

An import thing to remember relates to missing data: if any of your values is NA (not available; missing), these functions will return an NA. Either deal with your missing values beforehand (recommended) or add the `na.rm = TRUE` argument into any of the functions to ask R to ignore missing values. More discussion and examples around missing data can be found in Chapters 2 and 11.

```
mynumbers <- c(1, 2, NA)
sum(mynumbers)
```

```
## [1] NA
```

```
sum(mynumbers, na.rm = TRUE)
```

```
## [1] 3
```

Overall, R's unwillingness to implicitly average over observations with missing values should be considered helpful, not an unnecessary pain. If you don't know exactly where your missing values are, you might end up comparing the averages of different groups. So the `na.rm = TRUE` is fine to use if quickly exploring and cleaning data, or if you've already investigated missing values and are convinced the existing ones are representative. But it is rightfully not a default so get used to typing `na.rm = TRUE` when using these functions.

3.7 `select()` columns

The `select()` function can be used to choose, rename, or reorder columns of a tibble.

For the following `select()` examples, let's create a new tibble called `gbd_2rows` by taking the first 2 rows of `gbd_full` (just for shorter printing):

```
gbd_2rows <- gbd_full %>%
  slice(1:2)
```

```
gbd_2rows
```

```
## # A tibble: 2 x 5
##   cause                    year sex    income       deaths_millions
##   <chr>                   <dbl> <chr>  <chr>                  <dbl>
## 1 Communicable diseases    1990 Female High                    0.21
## 2 Communicable diseases    1990 Female Upper-Middle            1.150
```

Let's `select()` two of these columns:

```
gbd_2rows %>%
  select(cause, deaths_millions)
```

```
## # A tibble: 2 x 2
##   cause                 deaths_millions
##   <chr>                           <dbl>
## 1 Communicable diseases            0.21
## 2 Communicable diseases            1.150
```

We can also use `select()` to rename the columns we are choosing:

```
gbd_2rows %>%
  select(cause, deaths = deaths_millions)
```

```
## # A tibble: 2 x 2
##   cause                 deaths
##   <chr>                  <dbl>
## 1 Communicable diseases   0.21
## 2 Communicable diseases   1.150
```

There function `rename()` is similar to `select()`, but it keeps all variables whereas `select()` only kept the ones we mentioned:

```
gbd_2rows %>%
  rename(deaths = deaths_millions)
```

```
## # A tibble: 2 x 5
##   cause                    year sex    income       deaths
##   <chr>                   <dbl> <chr>  <chr>          <dbl>
## 1 Communicable diseases    1990 Female High            0.21
## 2 Communicable diseases    1990 Female Upper-Middle    1.150
```

`select()` can also be used to reorder the columns in your tibble. Moving columns around is not relevant in data analysis (as any of the functions we showed you above, as well as plotting, only look at the column names, and not their positions in the tibble), but it is useful for organising your tibble for easier viewing.

So if we use select like this:

```
gbd_2rows %>%
  select(year, sex, income, cause, deaths_millions)
```

```
## # A tibble: 2 x 5
##    year sex    income       cause                 deaths_millions
##   <dbl> <chr>  <chr>        <chr>                           <dbl>
## 1  1990 Female High         Communicable diseases            0.21
## 2  1990 Female Upper-Middle Communicable diseases            1.150
```

The columns are reordered.

If you want to move specific column(s) to the front of the tibble, do:

```
gbd_2rows %>%
  select(year, sex, everything())
```

```
## # A tibble: 2 x 5
##    year sex    cause                 income       deaths_millions
##   <dbl> <chr>  <chr>                 <chr>                  <dbl>
## 1  1990 Female Communicable diseases High                   0.21
## 2  1990 Female Communicable diseases Upper-Middle           1.150
```

And this is where the true power of `select()` starts to come out. In addition
to listing the columns explicitly (e.g., `mydata %>% select(year, cause...)`) there
are several special functions that can be used inside `select()`. These special
functions are called select helpers, and the first select helper we used is `every-
thing()`.

The most common select helpers are `starts_with()`, `ends_with()`, `contains()`,
`matches()` (but there are several others that may be useful to you, so press
F1 on `select()` for a full list, or search the web for more examples).

Let's say you can remember, whether the deaths column was called
`deaths_millions` or just `deaths` or `deaths_mil`, or maybe there are other columns
that include the word "deaths" that you want to `select()`:

```
gbd_2rows %>%
  select(starts_with("deaths"))
```

```
## # A tibble: 2 x 1
##   deaths_millions
##             <dbl>
## 1            0.21
## 2            1.150
```

Note how "deaths" needs to be quoted inside `starts_with()` - as it's a word to
look for, not the real name of a column/variable.

3.8   Reshaping data - long vs wide format

So far, all of the examples we've shown you have been using 'tidy' data. Data is 'tidy' when it is in long format: *each variable is in its own column*, and *each observation is in its own row*. This long format is efficient to use in data analysis and visualisation and can also be considered "computer readable".

But sometimes when presenting data in tables for humans to read, or when collecting data directly into a spreadsheet, it can be convenient to have data in a wide format. Data is 'wide' when *some or all of the columns are levels of a factor*. An example makes this easier to see.

```
gbd_wide <- read_csv("data/global_burden_disease_wide-format.csv")
gbd_long <- read_csv("data/global_burden_disease_cause-year-sex.csv")
```

TABLE 3.2: Global Burden of Disease data in human-readable wide format. This is not tidy data.

cause	Female_1990	Female_2017	Male_1990	Male_2017
Communicable diseases	7.30	4.91	8.06	5.47
Injuries	1.41	1.42	2.84	3.05
Non-communicable diseases	12.80	19.15	13.91	21.74

TABLE 3.3: Global Burden of Disease data in analysis-friendly long format. This is tidy data.

cause	year	sex	deaths_millions
Communicable diseases	1990	Female	7.30
Communicable diseases	2017	Female	4.91
Communicable diseases	1990	Male	8.06
Communicable diseases	2017	Male	5.47
Injuries	1990	Female	1.41
Injuries	2017	Female	1.42
Injuries	1990	Male	2.84
Injuries	2017	Male	3.05
Non-communicable diseases	1990	Female	12.80
Non-communicable diseases	2017	Female	19.15
Non-communicable diseases	1990	Male	13.91
Non-communicable diseases	2017	Male	21.74

Tables 3.3 and 3.2 contain the exact same information, but in long (tidy) and wide formats, respectively.

3.8.1 Pivot values from rows into columns (wider)

If we want to take the long data from 3.3 and put some of the numbers next to each other for easier visualisation, then `pivot_wider()` from the **tidyr** package is the function to do it. It means we want to send a variable into columns, and it needs just two arguments: the variable we want to become the new columns, and the variable where the values currently are.

```
gbd_long %>%
  pivot_wider(names_from = year, values_from = deaths_millions)
```

```
## # A tibble: 6 x 4
##   cause                      sex     `1990` `2017`
##   <chr>                      <chr>    <dbl>  <dbl>
## 1 Communicable diseases      Female    7.3    4.91
## 2 Communicable diseases      Male      8.06   5.47
## 3 Injuries                   Female    1.41   1.42
## 4 Injuries                   Male      2.84   3.05
## 5 Non-communicable diseases  Female   12.8   19.15
## 6 Non-communicable diseases  Male     13.91  21.74
```

This means we can quickly eyeball how the number of deaths has changed from 1990 to 2017 for each cause category and sex. Whereas if we wanted to quickly look at the difference in the number of deaths for females and males, we can change the `names_from =` argument from `= years` to `= sex`. Furthermore, we can also add a `mutate()` to calculate the difference:

```
gbd_long %>%
  pivot_wider(names_from = sex, values_from = deaths_millions) %>%
  mutate(Male - Female)
```

```
## # A tibble: 6 x 5
##   cause                      year Female  Male `Male - Female`
##   <chr>                     <dbl>  <dbl> <dbl>           <dbl>
## 1 Communicable diseases      1990   7.3   8.06           0.76
## 2 Communicable diseases      2017   4.91  5.47           0.5600
## 3 Injuries                   1990   1.41  2.84           1.430
## 4 Injuries                   2017   1.42  3.05           1.63
## 5 Non-communicable diseases  1990  12.8  13.91           1.110
## 6 Non-communicable diseases  2017  19.15 21.74           2.59
```

All of these differences are positive which means every year, more men die than women. Which make sense, as more boys are born than girls.

And what if we want to look at both `year` and `sex` at the same time, so to create Table 3.2 from Table 3.3? No problem, `pivot_wider()` can deal with multiple variables at the same time, `names_from = c(sex, year)`:

```
gbd_long %>%
  pivot_wider(names_from = c(sex, year), values_from = deaths_millions)
```

```
## # A tibble: 3 x 5
##   cause                      Female_1990 Female_2017 Male_1990 Male_2017
##   <chr>                            <dbl>       <dbl>     <dbl>     <dbl>
## 1 Communicable diseases              7.3        4.91      8.06      5.47
## 2 Injuries                          1.41        1.42      2.84      3.05
## 3 Non-communicable diseases         12.8       19.15     13.91     21.74
```

`pivot_wider()` has a few optional arguments that may be useful for you. For example, `pivot_wider(..., values_fill = 0)` can be used to fill empty cases (if you have any) with a value you specified. Or `pivot_wider(..., names_sep = ": ")` can be used to change the separator that gets put between the values (e.g., you may want "Female: 1990" instead of the default "Female_1990"). Remember that pressing F1 when your cursor is on a function opens it up in the Help tab where these extra options are listed.

3.8.2 Pivot values from columns to rows (longer)

The inverse of `pivot_wider()` is `pivot_longer()`. If you're lucky enough, your data comes from a proper database and is already in the long and tidy format. But if you do get landed with something that looks like Table 3.2, you'll need to know how to wrangle the variables currently spread across different columns into the tidy format (where each column is a variable, each row is an observation).

`pivot_longer()` can be a little bit more difficult to use as you need to describe all the columns to be collected using a `select_helper`. Run '?select_helpers and click on the first result in the Help tab for a reminder.

For example, here we want to collect all the columns that include the words Female or Male, the select helper for it is `matches("Female|Male")`:

```
gbd_wide %>%
  pivot_longer(matches("Female|Male"),
               names_to = "sex_year",
               values_to = "deaths_millions") %>%
  slice(1:6)
```

```
## # A tibble: 6 x 3
##   cause                 sex_year      deaths_millions
##   <chr>                 <chr>                   <dbl>
## 1 Communicable diseases Female_1990               7.3
## 2 Communicable diseases Female_2017              4.91
## 3 Communicable diseases Male_1990                8.06
## 4 Communicable diseases Male_2017                5.47
## 5 Injuries              Female_1990              1.41
## 6 Injuries              Female_2017              1.42
```

You're probably looking at the example above and thinking that's all nice and simple on this miniature example dataset, but how on earth will I figure this out on a real-world example. And you're right, we won't deny that `pivot_longer()` is one of the most technically complicated functions in this book, and it can take a lot of trial and error to get it to work. How to get started with your own `pivot_longer()` transformation is to first play with the `select()` function to make sure you are telling R exactly which columns to pivot into the longer format. For example, before working out the `pivot_longer()` code for the above example, we would figure this out first:

```
gbd_wide %>%
  select(matches("Female|Male"))
```

```
## # A tibble: 3 x 4
##    Female_1990 Female_2017 Male_1990 Male_2017
##          <dbl>       <dbl>     <dbl>     <dbl>
## 1          7.3        4.91      8.06      5.47
## 2         1.41        1.42      2.84      3.05
## 3         12.8       19.15     13.91     21.74
```

Then, knowing that `matches("Female|Male")` works as expected inside our little `select()` test, we can copy-paste it into `pivot_longer()` and add the `names_to` and `values_to` arguments. Both of these arguments are new column names that you can make up (in the above example, we are using "sex_year" and "deaths_millions").

3.8.3 `separate()` a column into multiple columns

While `pivot_longer()` did a great job fetching the different observations that were spread across multiple columns into a single one, it's still a combination of two variables - sex and year. We can use the `separate()` function to deal with that.

```
gbd_wide %>%
  # same pivot_longer as before
  pivot_longer(matches("Female|Male"),
               names_to = "sex_year",
               values_to = "deaths_millions") %>%
  separate(sex_year, into = c("sex", "year"), sep = "_", convert = TRUE)
```

```
## # A tibble: 12 x 4
##    cause                  sex    year deaths_millions
##    <chr>                  <chr> <int>           <dbl>
## 1 Communicable diseases  Female 1990             7.3
## 2 Communicable diseases  Female 2017             4.91
## 3 Communicable diseases  Male   1990             8.06
## 4 Communicable diseases  Male   2017             5.47
## 5 Injuries               Female 1990             1.41
```

```
## 6 Injuries                    Female 2017    1.42
## 7 Injuries                    Male   1990    2.84
## 8 Injuries                    Male   2017    3.05
## 9 Non-communicable diseases Female 1990   12.8
## 10 Non-communicable diseases Female 2017   19.15
## 11 Non-communicable diseases Male   1990   13.91
## 12 Non-communicable diseases Male   2017   21.74
```

We've also added `convert = TRUE` to `separate()` so `year` would get converted into a numeric variable. The combination of, e.g., "Female-1990" is a character variable, so after separating them both `sex` and `year` would still be classified as characters. But the `convert = TRUE` recognises that `year` is a number and will appropriately convert it into an integer.

3.9 `arrange()` rows

The `arrange()` function sorts rows based on the column(s) you want. By default, it arranges the tibble in ascending order:

```
gbd_long %>%
  arrange(deaths_millions) %>%
  # first 3 rows just for printing:
  slice(1:3)
```

```
## # A tibble: 3 x 4
##   cause      year sex    deaths_millions
##   <chr>     <dbl> <chr>            <dbl>
## 1 Injuries  1990 Female            1.41
## 2 Injuries  2017 Female            1.42
## 3 Injuries  1990 Male              2.84
```

For numeric variables, we can just use a - to sort in descending order:

```
gbd_long %>%
  arrange(-deaths_millions) %>%
  slice(1:3)
```

```
## # A tibble: 3 x 4
##   cause                      year sex    deaths_millions
##   <chr>                     <dbl> <chr>            <dbl>
## 1 Non-communicable diseases 2017 Male             21.74
## 2 Non-communicable diseases 2017 Female           19.15
## 3 Non-communicable diseases 1990 Male             13.91
```

The - doesn't work for categorical variables; they need to be put in `desc()` for arranging in descending order:

```
gbd_long %>%
  arrange(desc(sex)) %>%
  # printing rows 1, 2, 11, and 12
  slice(1,2, 11, 12)
```

```
## # A tibble: 4 x 4
##   cause                    year sex    deaths_millions
##   <chr>                   <dbl> <chr>            <dbl>
## 1 Communicable diseases    1990 Male              8.06
## 2 Communicable diseases    2017 Male              5.47
## 3 Non-communicable diseases 1990 Female          12.8
## 4 Non-communicable diseases 2017 Female          19.15
```

3.9.1   Factor levels

`arrange()` sorts characters alphabetically, whereas factors will be sorted by the order of their levels. Let's make the cause column into a factor:

```
gbd_factored <- gbd_long %>%
  mutate(cause = factor(cause))
```

When we first create a factor, its levels will be ordered alphabetically:

```
gbd_factored$cause %>% levels()
```

```
## [1] "Communicable diseases"     "Injuries"
## [3] "Non-communicable diseases"
```

But we can now use `fct_relevel()` inside `mutate()` to change the order of these levels:

```
gbd_factored <- gbd_factored %>%
  mutate(cause = cause %>%
           fct_relevel("Injuries"))

gbd_factored$cause %>% levels()
```

```
## [1] "Injuries"                  "Communicable diseases"
## [3] "Non-communicable diseases"
```

`fct_relevel()` brings the level(s) listed in it to the front.

So if we use `arrange()` on `gbd_factored`, the `cause` column will be sorted based on the order of its levels, not alphabetically. This is especially useful in two places:

- plotting - categorical variables that are characters will be ordered alphabetically (e.g., think barplots), regardless of whether the rows are arranged or not;

- statistical tests - the reference level of categorical variables that are characters is the alphabetically first (e.g., what the odds ratio is relative to).

However, making a character column into a factor gives us power to give its levels a non-alphabetical order, giving us control over plotting order or defining our reference levels for use in statistical tests.

3.10 Exercises

3.10.1 Exercise - `pivot_wider()`

Using the GBD dataset with variables `cause`, `year` (1990 and 2017 only), `sex` (as shown in Table 3.3):

```
gbd_long <- read_csv("data/global_burden_disease_cause-year-sex.csv")
```

Use `pivot_wider()` to put the `cause` variable into columns using the `deaths_millions` as values:

TABLE 3.4: Exercise: putting the cause variable into the wide format.

year	sex	Communicable diseases	Injuries	Non-communicable diseases
1990	Female	7.30	1.41	12.80
2017	Female	4.91	1.42	19.15
1990	Male	8.06	2.84	13.91
2017	Male	5.47	3.05	21.74

Solution

```
gbd_long = read_csv("data/global_burden_disease_cause-year-sex.csv")
gbd_long %>%
  pivot_wider(names_from = cause, values_from = deaths_millions)
```

3.10.2 Exercise - `group_by()`, `summarise()`

Read in the full GBD dataset with variables `cause`, `year`, `sex`, `income`, `deaths_millions`.

```
gbd_full = read_csv("data/global_burden_disease_cause-year-sex-income.csv")

glimpse(gbd_full)
```

```
## Rows: 168
## Columns: 5
## $ cause          <chr> "Communicable diseases", "Communicable diseases", "...
## $ year           <dbl> 1990, 1990, 1990, 1990, 1990, 1990, 1990, 1990, 199...
## $ sex            <chr> "Female", "Female", "Female", "Female", "Male", "Ma...
## $ income         <chr> "High", "Upper-Middle", "Lower-Middle", "Low", "Hig...
## $ deaths_millions <dbl> 0.21, 1.15, 4.43, 1.51, 0.26, 1.35, 4.73, 1.72, 0.2...
```

Year 2017 of this dataset was shown in Table 3.1, the full dataset has seven times as many observations as Table 3.1 since it includes information about multiple years: 1990, 1995, 2000, 2005, 2010, 2015, 2017.

Investigate these code examples:

```
summary_data1 <-
  gbd_full %>%
  group_by(year) %>%
  summarise(total_per_year = sum(deaths_millions))


## `summarise()` ungrouping output (override with `.groups` argument)


summary_data1


## # A tibble: 7 x 2
##     year total_per_year
##    <dbl>          <dbl>
## 1   1990          46.32
## 2   1995          48.91
## 3   2000          50.38
## 4   2005          51.25
## 5   2010          52.63
## 6   2015          54.62
## 7   2017          55.74


summary_data2 <-
  gbd_full %>%
  group_by(year, cause) %>%
  summarise(total_per_cause = sum(deaths_millions))


## `summarise()` regrouping output by 'year' (override with `.groups` argument)


summary_data2


## # A tibble: 21 x 3
## # Groups:   year [7]
##     year cause                      total_per_cause
##    <dbl> <chr>                                <dbl>
## 1   1990 Communicable diseases                15.36
## 2   1990 Injuries                              4.25
## 3   1990 Non-communicable diseases            26.71
## 4   1995 Communicable diseases                15.11
## 5   1995 Injuries                              4.53
## 6   1995 Non-communicable diseases            29.27
```

```
##   7   2000 Communicable diseases              14.81
##   8   2000 Injuries                            4.56
##   9   2000 Non-communicable diseases          31.01
##  10   2005 Communicable diseases              13.89
## # ... with 11 more rows
```

You should recognise that:

- `summary_data1` includes the total number of deaths per year.
- `summary_data2` includes the number of deaths per cause per year.
- `summary_data1 =` means we are creating a new tibble called `summary_data1` and saving (=) results into it. If `summary_data1` was a tibble that already existed, it would get overwritten.
- `gbd_full` is the data being sent to the `group_by()` and then `summarise()` functions.
- `group_by()` tells `summarise()` that we want aggregated results for each year.
- `summarise()` then creates a new variable called `total_per_year` that sums the deaths from each different observation (subcategory) together.
- Calling `summary_data1` on a separate line gets it printed.
- We then do something similar in `summary_data2`.

Compare the number of rows (observations) and number of columns (variables) of `gbd_full`, `summary_data1`, and `summary_data2`.

You should notice that: * `summary_data2` has exactly 3 times as many rows (observations) as `summary_data1`. Why? * `gbd_full` has 5 variables, whereas the summarised tibbles have 2 and 3. Which variables got dropped? How?

Answers

- `gbd_full` has 168 observations (rows),
- `summary_data1` has 7,
- `summary_data2` has 21.

`summary_data1` was grouped by year, therefore it includes a (summarised) value for each year in the original dataset. `summary_data2` was grouped by year and cause (Communicable diseases, Injuries, Non-communicable diseases), so it has 3 values for each year.

The columns a `summarise()` function returns are: variables listed in `group_by()` + variables created inside `summarise()` (e.g., in this case `deaths_peryear`). All others get aggregated.

3.10.3 Exercise - `full_join()`, `percent()`

For each cause, calculate its percentage to total deaths in each year.

Hint: Use `full_join()` on `summary_data1` and `summary_data2`, and then use `mutate()` to add a new column called `percentage`.

Example result for a single year:

```
## Joining, by = "year"
```

```
## # A tibble: 3 x 5
##     year total_per_year cause                    total_per_cause percentage
##    <dbl>          <dbl> <chr>                              <dbl> <chr>
## 1  1990          46.32 Communicable diseases              15.36 33.161%
## 2  1990          46.32 Injuries                            4.25 9.175%
## 3  1990          46.32 Non-communicable diseases          26.71 57.664%
```

Solution

```
library(scales)
full_join(summary_data1, summary_data2) %>%
  mutate(percentage = percent(total_per_cause/total_per_year))
```

3.10.4   Exercise - mutate(), summarise()

Instead of creating the two summarised tibbles and using a full_join(), achieve the same result as in the previous exercise with a single pipeline using sum-marise() and then mutate().

Hint: you have to do it the other way around, so group_by(year, cause) %>% summarise(...) first, then group_by(year) %>% mutate().

Bonus: select() columns year, cause, percentage, then pivot_wider() the cause variable using percentage as values.

Solution

```
gbd_full %>%
  # aggregate to deaths per cause per year using summarise()
  group_by(year, cause) %>%
  summarise(total_per_cause = sum(deaths_millions)) %>%
  # then add a column of yearly totals using mutate()
  group_by(year) %>%
  mutate(total_per_year = sum(total_per_cause)) %>%
  # add the percentage column
  mutate(percentage = percent(total_per_cause/total_per_year)) %>%
  # select the final variables for better vieweing
  select(year, cause, percentage) %>%
  pivot_wider(names_from = cause, values_from = percentage)
```

```
## `summarise()` regrouping output by 'year' (override with `.groups` argument)
```

```
## # A tibble: 7 x 4
## # Groups:   year [7]
##     year `Communicable diseases` Injuries `Non-communicable diseases`
##    <dbl> <chr>                   <chr>    <chr>
## 1  1990 33%                     9%       58%
## 2  1995 31%                     9%       60%
## 3  2000 29%                     9%       62%
## 4  2005 27%                     9%       64%
```

```
## 5   2010 24%              9%        67%
## 6   2015 20%              8%        72%
## 7   2017 19%              8%        73%
```

Note that your pipelines shouldn't be much longer than this, and we often save interim results into separate tibbles for checking (like we did with `summary_data1` and `summary_data2`, making sure the number of rows are what we expect and spot checking that the calculation worked as expected).

R doesn't do what you want it to do, it does what you ask it to do. Testing and spot checking is essential as you will make mistakes. We sure do.

Do not feel like you should be able to just bash out these clever pipelines without a lot of trial and error first.

3.10.5   Exercise - `filter()`, `summarise()`, `pivot_wider()`

Still working with `gbd_full`:

- Filter for 1990.

- Calculate the total number of deaths in the different income groups (High, Upper-Middle, Lower-Middle, Low). Hint: use `group_by(income)` and `summarise(new_column_name = sum(variable))`.

- Calculate the total number of deaths within each income group for males and females. Hint: this is as easy as adding , `sex` to `group_by(income)`.

- `pivot_wider()` the `income` column.

Solution

```
gbd_full %>%
  filter(year == 1990) %>%
  group_by(income, sex) %>%
  summarise(total_deaths = sum(deaths_millions)) %>%
  pivot_wider(names_from = income, values_from = total_deaths)
```

```
## `summarise()` regrouping output by 'income' (override with `.groups` argument)

## # A tibble: 2 x 5
##   sex     High   Low `Lower-Middle` `Upper-Middle`
##   <chr>  <dbl> <dbl>          <dbl>          <dbl>
## 1 Female 4.140  2.22           8.47           6.68
## 2 Male    4.46  2.57           9.83          7.950
```

4

Different types of plots

What I cannot create, I do not understand.
Richard Feynman

There are a few different plotting packages in R, but the most elegant and versatile one is **ggplot2**[1]. **gg** stands for **g**rammar of **g**raphics which means that we can make a plot by describing it one component at a time. In other words, we build a plot by adding layers to it.

This does not have to be many layers, the simplest `ggplot()` consists of just two components:

- the variables to be plotted;
- a geometrical object (e.g., point, line, bar, box, etc.).

`ggplot()` calls geometrical objects *geoms*.

Figure 4.1 shows some example steps for building a scatter plot, including changing its appearance ('theme') and faceting - an efficient way of creating separate plots for subgroups.

---

[1]The name of the package is **ggplot2**, but the function is called `ggplot()`. For everything you've ever wanted to know about the grammar of graphics in R, see Wickham (2016).

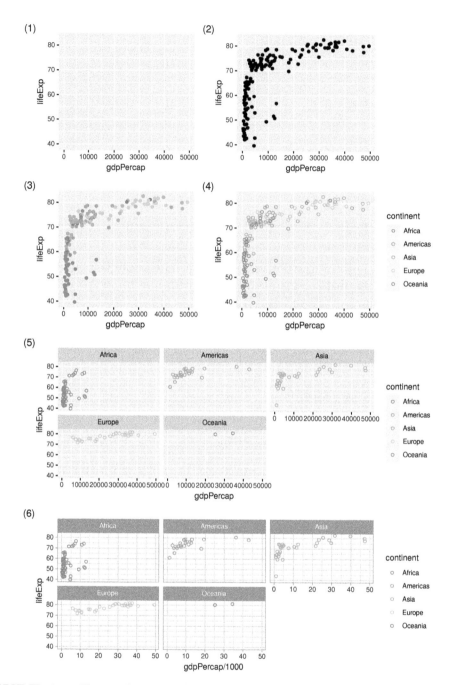

FIGURE 4.1: Example steps for building and modifying a ggplot. (1) Initialising the canvas and defining variables, (2) adding points, (3) colouring points by continent, (4) changing point type, (5) faceting, (6) changing the plot theme and the scale of the x variable.

4.1 Get the data

We are using the gapminder dataset (`https://www.gapminder.org/data`) that has been put into an R package by Bryan (2017) so we can load it with `library(gapminder)`.

```
library(tidyverse)
library(gapminder)

glimpse(gapminder)
```

```
## Rows: 1,704
## Columns: 6
## $ country   <fct> Afghanistan, Afghanistan, Afghanistan, Afghanistan, Afgha...
## $ continent <fct> Asia, Asia, Asia, Asia, Asia, Asia, Asia, Asia, Asia, Asi...
## $ year      <int> 1952, 1957, 1962, 1967, 1972, 1977, 1982, 1987, 1992, 199...
## $ lifeExp   <dbl> 28.801, 30.332, 31.997, 34.020, 36.088, 38.438, 39.854, 4...
## $ pop       <int> 8425333, 9240934, 10267083, 11537966, 13079460, 14880372,...
## $ gdpPercap <dbl> 779.4453, 820.8530, 853.1007, 836.1971, 739.9811, 786.113...
```

The dataset includes 1704 observations (rows) of 6 variables (columns: country, continent, year, lifeExp, pop, gdpPercap). `country`, `continent`, and `year` could be thought of as grouping variables, whereas lifeExp (life expectancy), pop (population), and gdpPercap (Gross Domestic Product per capita) are values.

The years in this dataset span 1952 to 2007 with 5-year intervals (so a total of 12 different years). It includes 142 countries from 5 continents (Asia, Europe, Africa, Americas, Oceania).

You can check that all of the numbers quoted above are correct with these lines:

```
library(tidyverse)
library(gapminder)
gapminder$year %>% unique()
gapminder$country %>% n_distinct()
gapminder$continent %>% unique()
```

Let's create a new shorter tibble called `gapdata2007` that only includes data for the year 2007.

```
gapdata2007 <- gapminder %>%
  filter(year == 2007)

gapdata2007
```

```
## # A tibble: 142 x 6
```

```
##       country     continent  year lifeExp         pop gdpPercap
##       <fct>       <fct>      <int>   <dbl>       <int>     <dbl>
##  1 Afghanistan Asia          2007    43.8    31889923      975.
##  2 Albania     Europe        2007    76.4     3600523     5937.
##  3 Algeria     Africa        2007    72.3    33333216     6223.
##  4 Angola      Africa        2007    42.7    12420476     4797.
##  5 Argentina   Americas      2007    75.3    40301927    12779.
##  6 Australia   Oceania       2007    81.2    20434176    34435.
##  7 Austria     Europe        2007    79.8     8199783    36126.
##  8 Bahrain     Asia          2007    75.6      708573    29796.
##  9 Bangladesh  Asia          2007    64.1   150448339     1391.
## 10 Belgium     Europe        2007    79.4    10392226    33693.
## # ... with 132 more rows
```

The new tibble - `gapdata2007` - now shows up in your Environment tab, whereas `gapminder` does not. Running `library(gapminder)` makes it available to use (so the funny line below is not necessary for any of the code in this chapter to work), but to have it appear in your normal Environment tab you'll need to run this funny looking line:

```
# loads the gapminder dataset from the package environment
# into your Global Environment
gapdata <- gapminder
```

Both `gapdata` and `gapdata2007` now show up in the Environment tab and can be clicked on/quickly viewed as usual.

4.2   Anatomy of ggplot explained

We will now explain the six steps shown in Figure 4.1. Note that you only need the first two to make a plot, the rest are just to show you further functionality and optional customisations.

(1) Start by defining the variables, e.g., `ggplot(aes(x = var1, y = var2))`:

```
gapdata2007 %>%
  ggplot(aes(x = gdpPercap, y = lifeExp))
```

This creates the first plot in Figure 4.1.

Although the above code is equivalent to:

```
ggplot(gapdata2007, aes(x = gdpPercap, y = lifeExp))
```

We tend to put the data first and then use the pipe (`%>%`) to send it to the `ggplot()` function. This becomes useful when we add further data wrangling functions between the data and the `ggplot()`. For example, our plotting pipelines often look like this:

```
data %>%
  filter(...) %>%
  mutate(...) %>%
  ggplot(aes(...)) +
  ...
```

The lines that come before the `ggplot()` function are piped, whereas from `ggplot()` onwards you have to use +. This is because we are now adding different layers and customisations to the same plot.

`aes()` stands for **aes**thetics - things we can see. Variables are always inside the `aes()` function, which in return is inside a `ggplot()`. Take a moment to appreciate the double closing brackets `))` - the first one belongs to `aes()`, the second one to `ggplot()`.

(2) Choose and add a geometrical object

Let's ask `ggplot()` to draw a point for each observation by adding `geom_point()`:

```
gapdata2007 %>%
  ggplot(aes(x = gdpPercap, y = lifeExp)) +
  geom_point()
```

We have now created the second plot in Figure 4.1, a scatter plot.

If we copy the above code and change just one thing - the x variable from `gdpPercap` to `continent` (which is a categorical variable) - we get what's called a strip plot. This means we are now plotting a continuous variable (`lifeExp`) against a categorical one (`continent`). But the thing to note is that the rest of the code stays exactly the same, all we did was change the x =.

```
gapdata2007 %>%
  ggplot(aes(x = continent, y = lifeExp)) +
  geom_point()
```

(3) specifying further variables inside `aes()`

Going back to the scatter plot (`lifeExp` vs `gdpPercap`), let's use `continent` to give the points some colour. We can do this by adding `colour = continent` inside the `aes()`:

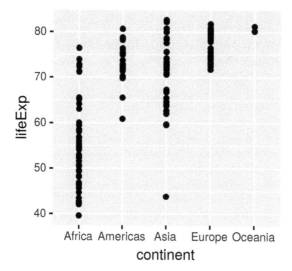

FIGURE 4.2: A strip plot using `geom_point()`.

```
gapdata2007 %>%
  ggplot(aes(x = gdpPercap, y = lifeExp, colour = continent)) +
  geom_point()
```

This creates the third plot in Figure 4.1. It uses the default colour scheme and will automatically include a legend. Still with just two lines of code (`ggplot(...)` + `geom_point()`).

(4) specifying aesthetics outside `aes()`

It is very important to understand the difference between including `ggplot` arguments inside or outside of the `aes()` function.

The main aesthetics (things we can see) are: **x**, **y**, **colour**, **fill**, **shape**, **size**, and any of these could appear inside or outside the `aes()` function. Press F1 on, e.g., `geom_point()`, to see the full list of aesthetics that can be used with this geom (this opens the Help tab). If F1 is hard to summon on your keyboard, type in and run `?geom_point`.

Variables (so columns of your dataset) have to be defined inside `aes()`. Whereas to apply a modification on everything, we can set an aesthetic to a constant value outside of `aes()`.

For example, Figure 4.3 shows a selection of the point shapes built into R. The default shape used by `geom_point()` is number 16.

To make all of the points in our figure hollow, let's set their shape to 1. We do this by adding `shape = 1` inside the `geom_point()`:

0 □ 1 ○ 2 △ 4 ✕ 8 ✳ 15 ■ 16 ● 17 ▲ 21 ⬤ 22 ▢ 23 ◇

FIGURE 4.3: A selection of shapes for plotting. Shapes 0, 1, and 2 are hollow, whereas for shapes 21, 22, and 23 we can define both a colour and a fill (for the shapes, colour is the border around the fill).

```
gapdata2007 %>%
    ggplot(aes(x = gdpPercap, y = lifeExp, colour = continent)) +
    geom_point(shape = 1)
```

This creates the fourth plot in Figure 4.1.

(5) From one plot to multiple with a single extra line

Faceting is a way to efficiently create the same plot for subgroups within the dataset. For example, we can separate each continent into its own facet by adding `facet_wrap(~continent)` to our plot:

```
gapdata2007 %>%
    ggplot(aes(x = gdpPercap, y = lifeExp, colour = continent)) +
    geom_point(shape = 1) +
    facet_wrap(~continent)
```

This creates the fifth plot in Figure 4.1. Note that we have to use the tilde (~) in `facet_wrap()`. There is a similar function called `facet_grid()` that will create a grid of plots based on two grouping variables, e.g., `facet_grid(var1~var2)`. Furthermore, facets are happy to quickly separate data based on a condition (so something you would usually use in a filter).

```
gapdata2007 %>%
    ggplot(aes(x = gdpPercap, y = lifeExp, colour = continent)) +
    geom_point(shape = 1) +
    facet_wrap(~pop > 50000000)
```

On this plot, the facet FALSE includes countries with a population less than 50 million people, and the facet TRUE includes countries with a population greater than 50 million people.

The tilde (~) in R denotes dependency. It is mostly used by statistical models to define dependent and explanatory variables and you will see it a lot in the second part of this book.

(6) Grey to white background - changing the theme

Overall, we can customise every single thing on a ggplot. Font type, colour, size or thickness or any lines or numbers, background, you name it. But a very

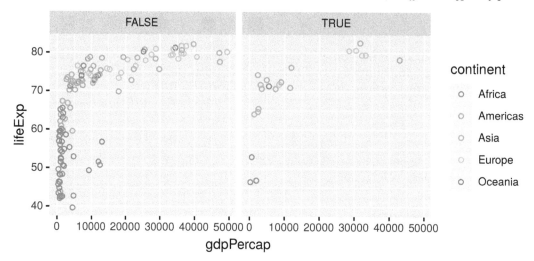

FIGURE 4.4: Using a filtering condition (e.g., population > 50 million) directly inside a `facet_wrap()`.

quick way to change the appearance of a ggplot is to apply a different theme. The signature ggplot theme has a light grey background and white grid lines (Figure 4.5).

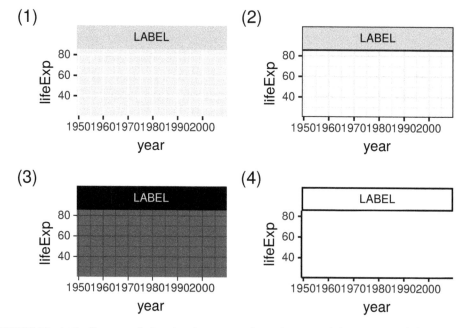

FIGURE 4.5: Some of the built-in ggplot themes (1) default (2) `theme_bw()`, (3) `theme_dark()`, (4) `theme_classic()`.

As a final step, we are adding `theme_bw()` ("background white") to give the plot a different look. We have also divided the gdpPercap by 1000 (making the units "thousands of dollars per capita"). Note that you can apply calculations directly on ggplot variables (so how we've done `x = gdpPercap/1000` here).

```
gapdata2007 %>%
  ggplot(aes(x = gdpPercap/1000, y = lifeExp, colour = continent)) +
  geom_point(shape = 1) +
  facet_wrap(~continent) +
  theme_bw()
```

This creates the last plot in Figure 4.1.

This is how `ggplot()` works - you can build a plot by adding or modifying things one by one.

4.3   Set your theme - grey vs white

If you find yourself always adding the same theme to your plot (i.e., we really like the `+ theme_bw()`), you can use `theme_set()` so your chosen theme is applied to every plot you draw:

```
theme_set(theme_bw())
```

In fact, we usually have these two lines at the top of every script:

```
library(tidyverse)
theme_set(theme_bw())
```

Furthermore, we can customise anything that appears in a `ggplot()` from axis fonts to the exact grid lines, and much more. That's what Chapter 5: Fine tuning plots is all about, but here we are focussing on the basic functionality and how different geoms work. But from now on,`+ theme_bw()` is automatically applied on everything we make.

4.4   Scatter plots/bubble plots

The ggplot anatomy (Section 4.2) covered both scatter and strip plots (both created with `geom_point()`). Another cool thing about this geom is that adding a size aesthetic makes it into a bubble plot. For example, let's size the points by population.

As you would expect from a "grammar of graphics plot", this is as simple as adding `size = pop` as an aesthetic:

```
gapdata2007 %>%
  ggplot(aes(x = gdpPercap/1000, y = lifeExp, size = pop)) +
  geom_point()
```

With increased bubble sizes, there is some overplotting, so let's make the points hollow (`shape = 1`) and slightly transparent (`alpha = 0.5`):

```
gapdata2007 %>%
  ggplot(aes(x = gdpPercap/1000, y = lifeExp, size = pop)) +
  geom_point(shape = 1, alpha = 0.5)
```

The resulting bubble plots are shown in Figure 4.6.

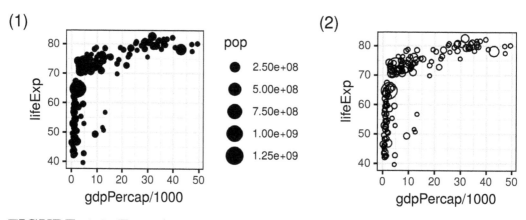

FIGURE 4.6: Turn the scatter plot from Figure 4.1:(2) to a bubble plot by (1) adding `size = pop` inside the `aes()`, (2) make the points hollow and transparent.

Alpha is an aesthetic to make geoms transparent, its values can range from 0 (invisible) to 1 (solid).

4.5   Line plots/time series plots

Let's plot the life expectancy in the United Kingdom over time (Figure 4.7):

```
gapdata %>%
  filter(country == "United Kingdom") %>%
  ggplot(aes(x = year, y = lifeExp)) +
  geom_line()
```

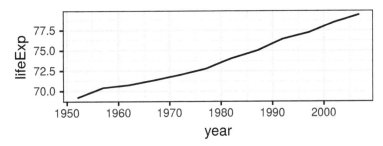

FIGURE 4.7: `geom_line()`- Life expectancy in the United Kingdom over time.

As a recap, the steps in the code above are:

- Send `gapdata` into a `filter()`;
- inside the `filter()`, our condition is `country == "United Kingdom"`;
- We initialise `ggplot()` and define our main variables: `aes(x = year, y = lifeExp)`;
- we are using a new geom - `geom_line()`.

This is identical to how we used `geom_point()`. In fact, by just changing `line` to `point` in the code above works - and instead of a continuous line you'll get a point at every 5 years as in the dataset.

But what if we want to draw multiple lines, e.g., for each country in the dataset? Let's send the whole dataset to `ggplot()` and `geom_line()`:

```
gapdata %>%
  ggplot(aes(x = year, y = lifeExp)) +
  geom_line()
```

The reason you see this weird zigzag in Figure 4.8 (1) is that, using the above code, `ggplot()` does not know which points to connect with which. Yes, you know you want a line for each country, but you haven't told it that. So for drawing multiple lines, we need to add a `group` aesthetic, in this case `group = country`:

```
gapdata %>%
  ggplot(aes(x = year, y = lifeExp, group = country)) +
  geom_line()
```

This code works as expected (Figure 4.8 (2)) - yes there is a lot of overplotting but that's just because we've included 142 lines on a single plot.

(1)   (2)

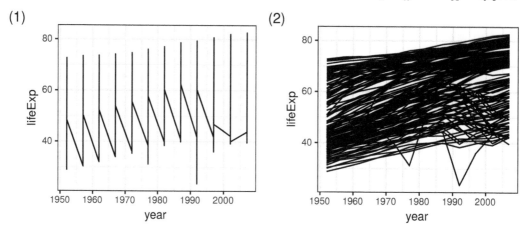

FIGURE 4.8: The 'zig-zag plot' is a common mistake: Using `geom_line()` (1) without a `group` specified, (2) after adding `group = country`.

4.5.1   Exercise

Follow the step-by-step instructions to transform Figure 4.8(2) into 4.9.

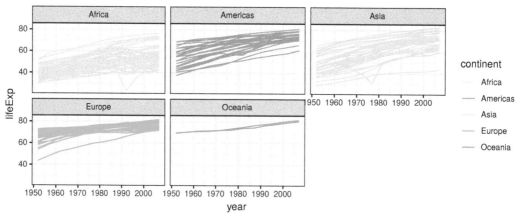

FIGURE 4.9: Lineplot exercise.

- Colour lines by continents: add `colour = continent` inside `aes()`;
- Continents on separate facets: `+ facet_wrap(~continent)`;
- Use a nicer colour scheme: `+ scale_colour_brewer(palette = "Paired")`.

4.6   Bar plots

There are two geoms for making bar plots - `geom_col()` and `geom_bar()` and the examples below will illustrate when to use which one. In short: if your data is already summarised or includes values for y (height of the bars), use `geom_col()`. If, however, you want `ggplot()` to count up the number of rows in your dataset, use `geom_bar()`. For example, with patient-level data (each row is a patient) you'll probably want to use `geom_bar()`, with data that is already somewhat aggregated, you'll use `geom_col()`. There is no harm in trying one, and if it doesn't work, trying the other.

4.6.1 Summarised data

- `geom_col()` requires two variables `aes(x = , y = )`
- x is categorical, y is continuous (numeric)

Let's plot the life expectancies in 2007 in these three countries:

```
gapdata2007 %>%
    filter(country %in% c("United Kingdom", "France", "Germany")) %>%
    ggplot(aes(x = country, y = lifeExp)) +
    geom_col()
```

This gives us Figure 4.10:1. We have also created another cheeky one using the same code but changing the scale of the y axis to be more dramatic (Figure 4.10:2).

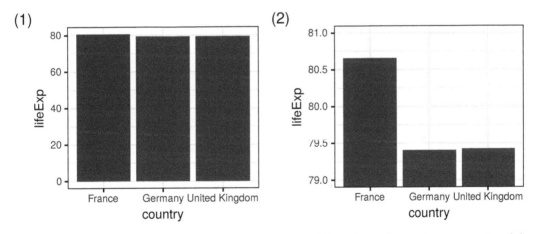

FIGURE 4.10: Bar plots using `geom_col()`: (1) using the code example, (2) same plot but with `+ coord_cartesian(ylim=c(79, 81))` to manipulate the scale into something a lot more dramatic.

4.6.2 Countable data

- `geom_bar()` requires a single variable `aes(x = )`
- this x should be a categorical variable

- `geom_bar()` then counts up the number of observations (rows) for this variable and plots them as bars.

Our `gapdata2007` tibble has a row for each country (see end of Section 4.1 to remind yourself). Therefore, if we use the `count()` function on the `continent` variable, we are counting up the number of countries on each continent (in this dataset[2]):

```
gapdata2007 %>%
  count(continent)
```

```
## # A tibble: 5 x 2
##    continent       n
##    <fct>       <int>
## 1 Africa         52
## 2 Americas       25
## 3 Asia           33
## 4 Europe         30
## 5 Oceania         2
```

So `geom_bar()` basically runs the `count()` function and plots it (see how the bars on Figure 4.11 are the same height as the values from `count(continent)`).

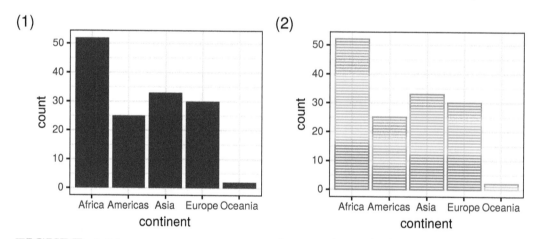

FIGURE 4.11: `geom_bar()` counts up the number of observations for each group. (1) `gapdata2007 %>% ggplot(aes(x = continent)) + geom_bar()`, (2) same + a little bit of magic to reveal the underlying data.

The first barplot in Figure 4.11 is produced with just this:

```
gapdata2007 %>%
  ggplot(aes(x = continent)) +
  geom_bar()
```

---

[2]The number of countries in this dataset is 142, whereas the United Nations have 193 member states.

Whereas on the second one, we've asked `geom_bar()` to reveal the components (countries) in a colourful way:

```
gapdata2007 %>%
  ggplot(aes(x = continent, colour = country)) +
  geom_bar(fill = NA) +
  theme(legend.position = "none")
```

We have added `theme(legend.position = "none")` to remove the legend - it includes all 142 countries and is not very informative in this case. We're only including the colours for a bit of fun.

We're also removing the fill by setting it to NA (`fill = NA`). Note how we defined `colour = country` inside the `aes()` (as it's a variable), but we put the fill inside `geom_bar()` as a constant. This was explained in more detail in steps (3) and (4) in the ggplot anatomy Section (4.2).

4.6.3 colour vs fill

Figure 4.11 also reveals the difference between a colour and a fill. Colour is the border around a geom, whereas fill is inside it. Both can either be set based on a variable in your dataset (this means `colour =` or `fill =` needs to be inside the `aes()` function), or they could be set to a fixed colour.

R has an amazing knowledge of colour. In addition to knowing what is "white", "yellow", "red", "green" etc. (meaning we can simply do `geom_bar(fill = "green")`), it also knows what "aquamarine", "blanchedalmond", "coral", "deeppink", "lavender", "deepskyblue" look like (amongst many many others; search the internet for "R colours" for a full list).

We can also use Hex colour codes, for example, `geom bar(fill = "#FF0099")` is a very pretty pink. Every single colour in the world can be represented with a Hex code, and the codes are universally known by most plotting or image making programmes. Therefore, you can find Hex colour codes from a lot of places on the internet, or `https://www.color-hex.com` just to name one.

4.6.4 Proportions

Whether using `geom_bar()` or `geom_col()`, we can use fill to display proportions within bars. Furthermore, sometimes it's useful to set the x value to a constant - to get everything plotted together rather than separated by a variable. So we are using `aes(x = "Global", fill = continent)`. Note that "Global" could be any word - since it's quoted `ggplot()` won't go looking for it in the dataset (Figure 4.12):

```
gapdata2007 %>%
  ggplot(aes(x = "Global", fill = continent)) +
  geom_bar()
```

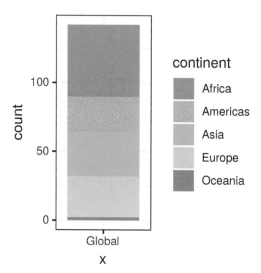

FIGURE 4.12: Number of countries in the gapminder datatset with proportions using the `fill = continent` aesthetic.

There are more examples of bar plots in Chapter 8.

4.6.5   Exercise

Create Figure 4.13 of life expectancies in European countries (year 2007).

Hints:

- If `geom_bar()` doesn't work try `geom_col()` or vice versa.
- `coord_flip()` to make the bars horizontal (it flips the `x` and `y` axes).
- `x = country` gets the country bars plotted in alphabetical order, use `x = fct_reorder(country, lifeExp)` still inside the `aes()` to order the bars by their `lifeExp` values. Or try one of the other variables (`pop`, `gdpPercap`) as the second argument to `fct_reorder()`.
- when using `fill = NA`, you also need to include a colour; we're using `colour = "deepskyblue"` inside the `geom_col()`.

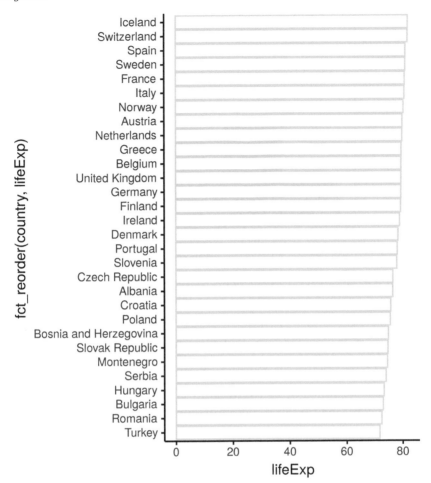

FIGURE 4.13: Barplot exercise. Life expectancies in European countries in year 2007 from the gapminder dataset.

4.7 Histograms

A histogram displays the distribution of values within a continuous variable. In the example below, we are taking the life expectancy (`aes(x = lifeExp)`) and telling the histogram to count the observations up in "bins" of 10 years (`geom_histogram(binwidth = 10)`, Figure 4.14):

```
gapdata2007 %>%
  ggplot(aes(x = lifeExp)) +
  geom_histogram(binwidth = 10)
```

We can see that most countries in the world have a life expectancy of ~70-80 years (in 2007), and that the distribution of life expectancies globally is not nor-

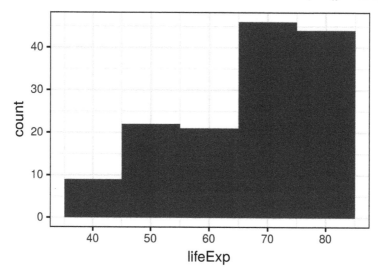

FIGURE 4.14: `geom_histogram()` - The distribution of life expectancies in different countries around the world in year 2007.

mally distributed. Setting the binwidth is optional, using just `geom_histogram()` works well too - by default, it will divide your data into 30 bins.

There are more examples of histograms in Chapter 6. There are two other geoms that are useful for plotting distributions: `geom_density()` and `geom_freqpoly()`.

4.8   Box plots

Box plots are our go to method for quickly visualising summary statistics of a continuous outcome variable (such as life expectancy in the gapminder dataset, Figure 4.15).

Box plots include:

- the median (middle line in the box)
- inter-quartile range (IQR, top and bottom parts of the boxes - this is where 50% of your data is)
- whiskers (the black lines extending to the lowest and highest values that are still within 1.5*IQR)
- outliers (any observations out with the whiskers)

```
gapdata2007 %>%
  ggplot(aes(x = continent, y = lifeExp)) +
  geom_boxplot()
```

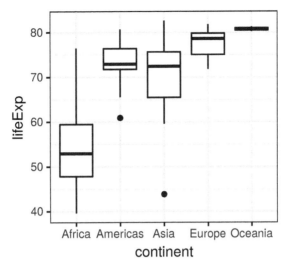

FIGURE 4.15: geom_boxplot() - Boxplots of life expectancies within each continent in year 2007.

4.9   Multiple geoms, multiple aes()

One of the coolest things about ggplot() is that we can plot multiple geoms on top of each other!

Let's add individual data points on top of the box plots:

```
gapdata2007 %>%
  ggplot(aes(x = continent, y = lifeExp)) +
  geom_boxplot() +
  geom_point()
```

This makes Figure 4.16(1).

The only thing we've changed in (2) is replacing geom_point() with geom_jitter() - this spreads the points out to reduce overplotting.

But what's really exciting is the difference between (3) and (4) in Figure 4.16. Spot it!

```
# (3)
gapdata2007 %>%
  ggplot(aes(x = continent, y = lifeExp, colour = continent)) +
  geom_boxplot() +
  geom_jitter()

# (4)
gapdata2007 %>%
```

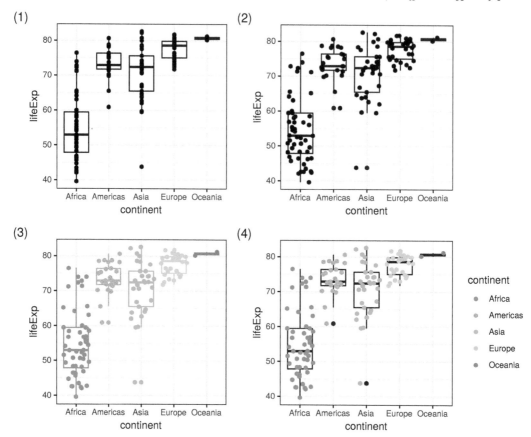

FIGURE 4.16: Multiple geoms together. (1) `geom_boxplot() + geom_point()`, (2) `geom_boxplot() + geom_jitter()`, (3) colour aesthetic inside `ggplot(aes())`, (4) colour aesthetic inside `geom_jitter(aes())`.

```
ggplot(aes(x = continent, y = lifeExp)) +
geom_boxplot() +
geom_jitter(aes(colour = continent))
```

This is new: `aes()` inside a geom, not just at the top! In the code for (4) you can see `aes()` in two places - at the top and inside the `geom_jitter()`. And `colour = continent` was only included in the second `aes()`. This means that the jittered points get a colour, but the box plots will be drawn without (so just black). This is exactly* what we see on 4.16.

*Nerd alert: the variation added by `geom_jitter()` is random, which means that when you recreate the same plots the points will appear in slightly different locations to ours. To make identical ones, add `position = position_jitter(seed = 1)` inside `geom_jitter()`.

4.9.1   Worked example - three geoms together

Let's combine three geoms by including text labels on top of the box plot + points from above.

We are creating a new tibble called `label_data` filtering for the maximum life expectancy countries at each continent (`group_by(continent)`):

```
label_data <- gapdata2007 %>%
  group_by(continent) %>%
  filter(lifeExp == max(lifeExp)) %>%
  select(country, continent, lifeExp)

# since we filtered for lifeExp == max(lifeExp)
# these are the maximum life expectancy countries at each continent:
label_data
```

```
## # A tibble: 5 x 3
## # Groups:   continent [5]
##   country   continent lifeExp
##   <fct>     <fct>        <dbl>
## 1 Australia Oceania       81.2
## 2 Canada    Americas      80.7
## 3 Iceland   Europe        81.8
## 4 Japan     Asia          82.6
## 5 Reunion   Africa        76.4
```

The first two geoms are from the previous example (`geom_boxplot()` and `geom_jitter()`). Note that `ggplot()` plots them in the order they are in the code - so box plots at the bottom, jittered points on the top. We are then adding `geom_label()` with its own data option (`data = label_data`) as well as a new aesthetic (`aes(label = country)`, Figure 4.17):

```
gapdata2007 %>%
  ggplot(aes(x = continent, y = lifeExp)) +
  # First geom - boxplot
  geom_boxplot() +
  # Second geom - jitter with its own aes(colour = )
  geom_jitter(aes(colour = continent)) +
  # Third geom - label, with its own dataset (label_data) and aes(label = )
  geom_label(data = label_data, aes(label = country))
```

A few suggested experiments to try with the 3-geom plot code above:

- remove `data = label_data,` from `geom_label()` and you'll get all 142 labels (so it will plot a label for the whole `gapdata2007` dataset);
- change from `geom_label()` to `geom_text()` - it works similarly but doesn't have the border and background behind the country name;
- change `label = country` to `label = lifeExp`, this plots the maximum value, rather than the country name.

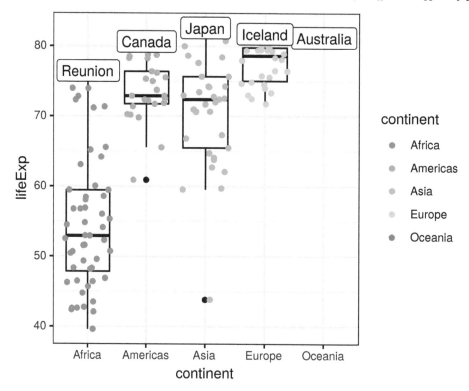

FIGURE 4.17: Three geoms together on a single plot: `geom_boxplot()`, `geom_jitter()`, and `geom_label()`.

4.10 All other types of plots

In this chapter we have introduced some of the most common geoms, as well as explained how `ggplot()` works. In fact, ggplot has 56 different geoms for you to use; see its documentation for a full list: `https://ggplot2.tidyverse.org`.

With the ability of combining multiple geoms together on the same plot, the possibilities really are endless. Furthermore, the plotly Graphic Library (`https://plot.ly/ggplot2/`) can make some of your ggplots interactive, meaning you can use your mouse to hover over the point or zoom and subset interactively.

The two most important things to understand about `ggplot()` are:

- Variables (columns in your dataset) need to be inside `aes()`;
- `aes()` can be both at the top - `data %>% ggplot(aes())` - as well as inside a geom (e.g., `geom_point(aes())`). This distinction is useful when combining multiple geoms. All your geoms will "know about" the top-level `aes()` variables, but including `aes()` variables inside a specific geom means it only applies to that one.

4.11   Solutions

Solution to Exercise 4.5.1:

```
library(tidyverse)
library(gapminder)

gapminder %>%
  ggplot(aes(x       = year,
             y       = lifeExp,
             group   = country,
             colour  = continent)) +
  geom_line() +
  facet_wrap(~continent) +
  theme_bw() +
  scale_colour_brewer(palette = "Paired")
```

Solution to Exercise 4.6.5:

```
library(tidyverse)
library(gapminder)

gapminder %>%
  filter(year == 2007) %>%
  filter(continent == "Europe") %>%
  ggplot(aes(x = fct_reorder(country, lifeExp), y = lifeExp)) +
  geom_col(colour = "deepskyblue", fill = NA) +
  coord_flip() +
  theme_classic()
```

4.12   Extra: Advanced examples

There are two examples of how just a few lines of `ggplot()` code and the basic geoms introduced in this chapter can be used to make very different things. Let your imagination fly free when using `ggplot()`!

Figure 4.18 shows how the life expectancies in European countries have increased by plotting a square (`geom_point(shape = 15)`) for each observation (year) in the dataset.

```
gapdata %>%
  filter(continent == "Europe") %>%
  ggplot(aes(y       = fct_reorder(country, lifeExp, .fun=max),
```

```
              x      = lifeExp,
           colour = year)) +
geom_point(shape = 15, size = 2) +
scale_colour_distiller(palette = "Greens", direction = 1) +
theme_bw()
```

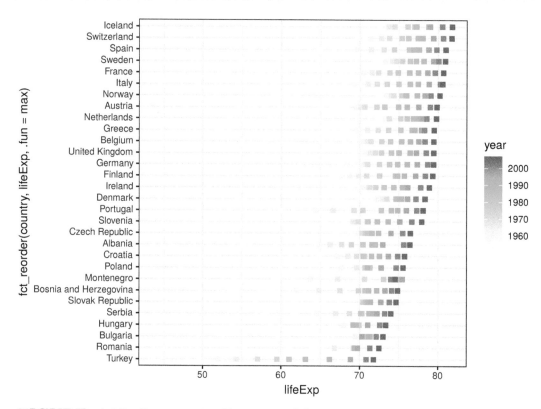

FIGURE 4.18: Increase in European life expectancies over time. Using `fct_reorder()` to order the countries on the y-axis by life expectancy (rather than alphabetically which is the default).

In Figure 4.19, we're using `group_by(continent)` followed by `mutate(country_number = seq_along(country))` to create a new column with numbers 1, 2, 3, etc., for countries within continents. We are then using these as `y` coordinates for the text labels (`geom_text(aes(y = country_number...)`).

```
gapdata2007 %>%
  group_by(continent) %>%
  mutate(country_number = seq_along(country)) %>%
  ggplot(aes(x = continent)) +
  geom_bar(aes(colour = continent), fill = NA, show.legend = FALSE) +
  geom_text(aes(y = country_number, label = country), vjust = 1)+
  geom_label(aes(label = continent), y = -1) +
  theme_void()
```

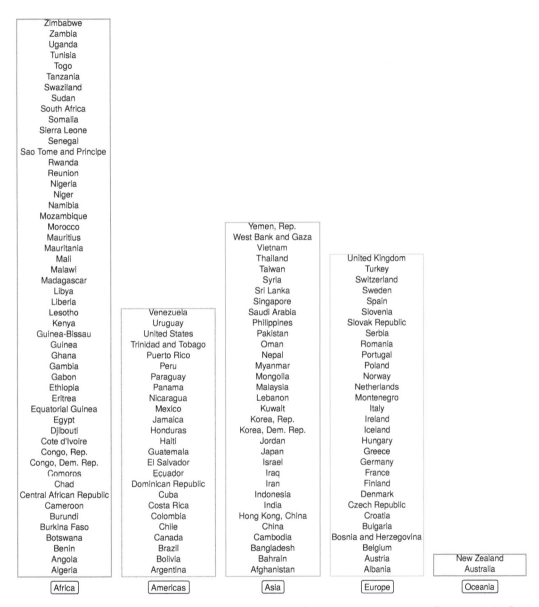

FIGURE 4.19: List of countries on each continent as in the gapminder dataset.

5

Fine tuning plots

5.1 Get the data

We can save a `ggplot()` object into a variable (we usually call it `p` but it can be any name). This then appears in the Environment tab. To plot it it needs to be recalled on a separate line to get drawn (Figure 5.1). Saving a plot into a variable allows us to modify it later (e.g., `p + theme_bw()`).

```
library(gapminder)
library(tidyverse)

p0 <- gapminder %>%
   filter(year == 2007) %>%
   ggplot(aes(y = lifeExp, x = gdpPercap, colour = continent)) +
   geom_point(alpha = 0.3) +
   theme_bw() +
   geom_smooth(method = "lm", se = FALSE) +
   scale_colour_brewer(palette = "Set1")

p0
```

5.2 Scales

5.2.1 Logarithmic

Transforming an axis to a logarithmic scale can be done by adding on `scale_x_log10()`:

```
p1 <- p0 + scale_x_log10()
```

`scale_x_log10()` and `scale_x_log10()` are shortcuts for the base-10 logarithmic transformation of an axis. The same could be achieved by using, e.g., `scale_x_continuous(trans = "log10")`. The latter can take a selection of options,

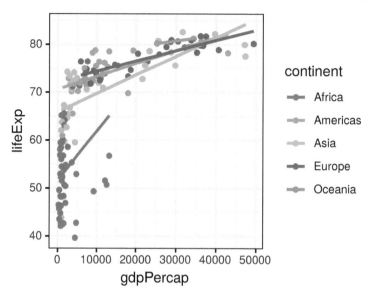

FIGURE 5.1: p0: Starting plot for the examples in this chapter.

namely `"reverse"`, `"log2"`, or `"sqrt"`. Check the Help tab for `scale_continuous()` or look up its online documentation for a full list.

5.2.2 Expand limits

A quick way to expand the limits of your plot is to specify the value you want to be included:

```
p2 <- p0 + expand_limits(y = 0)
```

Or two values for extending to both sides of the plot:

```
p3 <- p0 + expand_limits(y = c(0, 100))
```

By default, `ggplot()` adds some padding around the included area (see how the scale doesn't start from 0, but slightly before). This ensures points on the edges don't get overlapped with the axes, but in some cases - especially if you've already expanded the scale, you might want to remove this extra padding. You can remove this padding with the `expand` argument:

```
p4 <- p0 +
  expand_limits(y = c(0, 100)) +
  coord_cartesian(expand = FALSE)
```

We are now using a new library - **patchwork** - to print all 4 plots together

(Figure 5.2). Its syntax is very simple - it allows us to add ggplot objects together. (Trying to do `p1 + p2` without loading the **patchwork** package will not work, R will say "Error: Don't know how to add p2 to a plot".)

```
library(patchwork)
p1 + p2 + p3 + p4 + plot_annotation(tag_levels = "1", tag_prefix = "p")
```

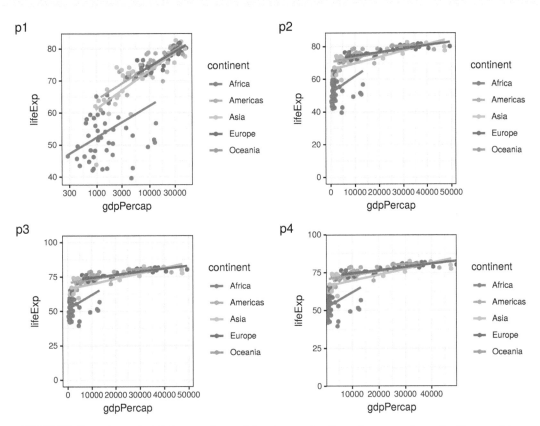

FIGURE 5.2: p1: Using a logarithmic scale for the x axis. p2: Expanding the limits of the y axis to include 0. p3: Expanding the limits of the y axis to include 0 and 100. p4: Removing extra padding around the limits.

5.2.3   Zoom in

```
p5 <- p0 +
  coord_cartesian(ylim = c(70, 85), xlim = c(20000, 40000))
```

5.2.4   Exercise

How is this one different to the previous (Figure 5.3)?

```
p6 <- p0 +
  scale_y_continuous(limits = c(70, 85)) +
  scale_x_continuous(limits = c(20000, 40000))
```

Answer: the first one zooms in, still retaining information about the excluded points when calculating the linear regression lines. The second one removes the data (as the warnings say), calculating the linear regression lines only for the visible points.

```
p5 + labs(tag = "p5") + p6 + labs(tag = "p6")
```

```
## Warning: Removed 114 rows containing non-finite values (stat_smooth).
```

```
## Warning: Removed 114 rows containing missing values (geom_point).
```

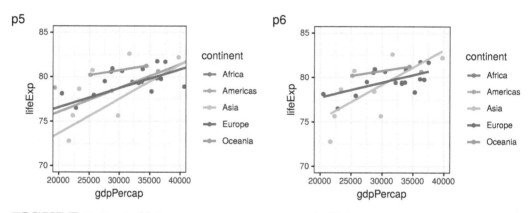

FIGURE 5.3: p5: Using `coord_cartesian()` vs p6: Using `scale_x_continuous()` and `scale_y_continuous()` for setting the limits of plot axes.

Preivously we used **patchwork**'s `plot_annotation()` function to create our multiplot tags. Since our exmaples no longer start the count from 1, we're using `ggplot()`'s tags instead, e.g., `labs(tag = "p5")`. The `labs()` function iwill be covered in more detail later in this chapter.

5.2.5   Axis ticks

`ggplot()` does a good job deciding how many and which values include on the axis (e.g., 70/75/80/85 for the y axes in Figure 5.3). But sometimes you'll want to specify these, for example, to indicate threshold values or a maximum (Figure 5.4). We can do so by using the `breaks` argument:

```
# calculating the maximum value to be included in the axis breaks:
max_value = gapminder %>%
  filter(year == 2007) %>%
```

```
  summarise(max_lifeExp = max(lifeExp)) %>%
  pull(max_lifeExp) %>%
  round(1)

# using scale_y_continuous(breaks = ...):
p7 <-  p0 +
  coord_cartesian(ylim = c(0, 100), expand = 0) +
  scale_y_continuous(breaks = c(18, 50, max_value))

# we may also include custom labels for our breaks:
p8 <-  p0 +
  coord_cartesian(ylim = c(0, 100), expand = 0) +
  scale_y_continuous(breaks = c(18, 50, max_value), labels = c("Adults", "50", "MAX"))

p7 + labs(tag = "p7") + p8 + labs(tag = "p8")
```

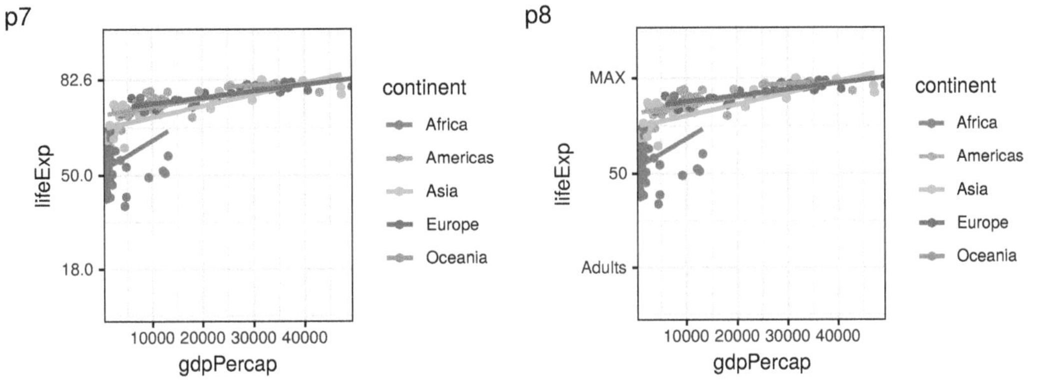

FIGURE 5.4: p7: Specifiying y axis breaks. p8: Adding custom labels for our breaks.

5.3   Colours

5.3.1   Using the Brewer palettes:

The easiest way to change the colour palette of your `ggplot()` is to specify a Brewer palette (Harrower and Brewer (2003)):

```
p9 <- p0 +
  scale_color_brewer(palette = "Paired")
```

Note that `http://colorbrewer2.org/` also has options for *Colourblind safe* and *Print friendly.*

5.3.2 Legend title

`scale_colour_brewer()` is also a convenient place to change the legend title (Figure 5.5):

```
p10 <- p0 +
  scale_color_brewer("Continent - \n one of 5", palette = "Paired")
```

Note the `\n` inside the new legend title - new line.

```
p9 + labs(tag = "p9") + p10 + labs(tag = "p10")
```

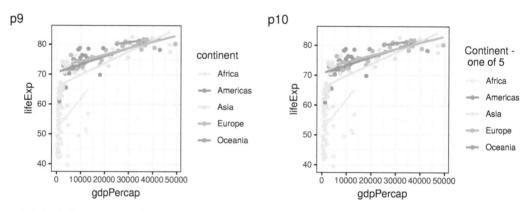

FIGURE 5.5: p9: Choosing a Brewer palette for your colours. p10: Changing the legend title.

5.3.3 Choosing colours manually

R also knows the names of many colours, so we can use words to specify colours:

```
p11 <- p0 +
  scale_color_manual(values = c("red", "green", "blue", "purple", "pink"))
```

The same function can also be used to use HEX codes for specifying colours:

```
p12 <- p0 +
  scale_color_manual(values = c("#8dd3c7", "#ffffb3", "#bebada",
                                "#fb8072", "#80b1d3"))
```

```
p11 + labs(tag = "p11") + p12 + labs(tag = "p12")
```

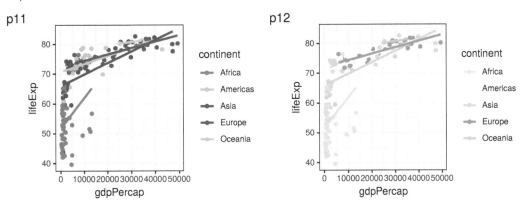

FIGURE 5.6: Colours can also be specified using words (`"red"`, `"green"`, etc.), or HEX codes (`"#8dd3c7"`, `"#ffffb3"`, etc.).

5.4 Titles and labels

We've been using the `labs(tag = )` function to add tags to plots. But the `labs()` function can also be used to modify axis labels, or to add a title, subtitle, or a caption to your plot (Figure 5.7):

```
p13 <- p0 +
  labs(x = "Gross domestic product per capita",
       y = "Life expectancy",
       title = "Health and economics",
       subtitle = "Gapminder dataset, 2007",
       caption = Sys.Date(),
       tag = "p13")

p13
```

5.4.1 Annotation

In the previous chapter, we showed how use `geom_text()` and `geom_label()` to add text elements to a plot. Using geoms make sense when the values are based on data and variables mapped in `aes()`. They are efficient for including multiple pieces of text or labels on your data. For 'hand' annotating a plot, the `annotate()` function makes more sense, as you can quickly insert the type, location and label of your annotation (Figure 5.8):

```
p14 <- p0 +
  annotate("text",
           x = 25000,
```

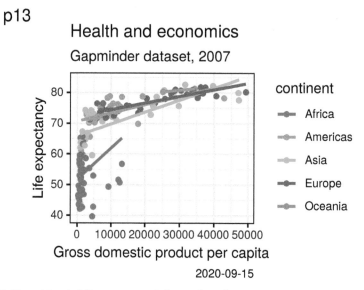

FIGURE 5.7: p13: Adding on a title, subtitle, caption using `labs()`.

```
            y = 50,
            label = "No points here!")



p15 <- p0 +
  annotate("label",
           x = 25000,
           y = 50,
           label = "No points here!")



p16 <- p0 +
  annotate("label",
           x = 25000,
           y = 50,
           label = "No points here!",
           hjust = 0)



p14 + labs(tag = "p14") + (p15 + labs(tag = "p15"))/ (p16 + labs(tag = "p16"))
```

`hjust` stands for horizontal justification. Its default value is 0.5 (see how the label was centred at 25,000 - our chosen x location), 0 means the label goes to the right from 25,000, 1 would make it end at 25,000.

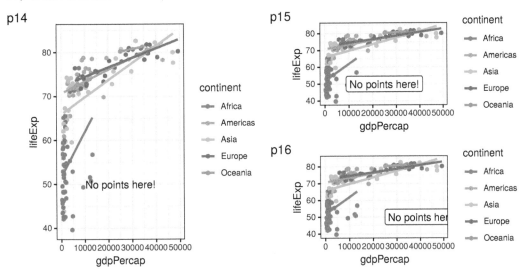

FIGURE 5.8: p14: `annotate("text", ...)` to quickly add a text on your plot. p15: `annotate("label")` is similar but draws a box around your text (making it a label). p16: Using `hjust` to control the horizontal justification of the annotation.

5.4.2 Annotation with a superscript and a variable

This is an advanced example on how to annotate your plot with something that has a superscipt and is based on a single value read in from a variable (Figure 5.9):

```r
# a value we made up for this example
# a real analysis would get it from the linear model object
fit_glance <- tibble(r.squared = 0.7693465)


plot_rsquared <- paste0(
  "R^2 == ",
  fit_glance$r.squared %>% round(2))


p17 <- p0 +
  annotate("text",
           x = 25000,
           y = 50,
           label = plot_rsquared, parse = TRUE,
           hjust = 0)

p17 + labs(tag = "p17")
```

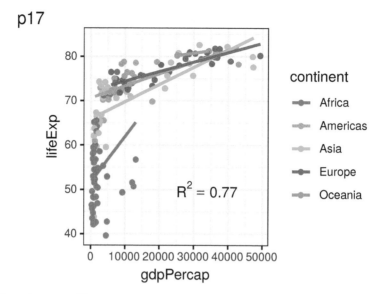

FIGURE 5.9: p17: Using a superscript in your plot annotation.

5.5 Overall look - `theme()`

And finally, everything else on a plot - from font to background to the space between facets, can be changed using the `theme()` function. As you saw in the previous chapter, in addition to its default grey background, `ggplot2` also comes with a few built-in themes, namely, `theme_bw()` or `theme_classic()`. These produce good looking plots that may already be publication ready. But if we do decide to tweak them, then the main `theme()` arguments we use are `axis.text`, `axis.title`, and `legend.position`.[1] Note that all of these go inside the `theme()`, and that the `axis.text` and `axis.title` arguments are usually followed by `= element_text()` as shown in the examples below.

5.5.1 Text size

The way the `axis.text` and `axis.title` arguments of `theme()` work is that if you specify `.x` or `.y` it gets applied on that axis alone. But not specifying these, applies the change on both. Both the `angle` and `vjust` (vertical justification) options can be useful if your axis text doesn't fit well and overlaps. It doesn't usually make sense to change the colour of the font to anything other than `"black"`, we are using green and red here to indicate which parts of the plot get changed with each line (Figure 5.10).

---

[1]To see a full list of possible arguments to `theme()`, navigate to it in the Help tab or find its online documentation at `https://ggplot2.tidyverse.org/`.

```
p18 <-  p0 +
  theme(axis.text.y = element_text(colour = "green", size = 14),
        axis.text.x = element_text(colour = "red",  angle = 45, vjust = 0.5),
        axis.title  = element_text(colour = "blue", size = 16)
        )

p18 + labs(tag = "p18")
```

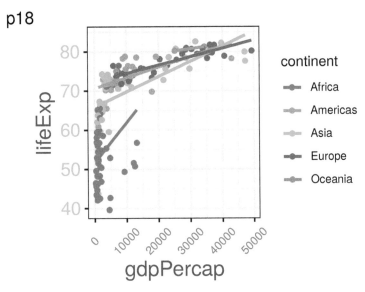

FIGURE 5.10: p18: Using `axis.text` and `axis.title` within `theme()` to tweak the appearance of your plot, including font size and angle. Coloured font is used to indicate which part of the code was used to change each element.

5.5.2 Legend position

The position of the legend can be changed using the `legend.position` argument within `theme()`. It can be positioned using the following words: `"right"`, `"left"`, `"top"`, `"bottom"`. Or to remove the legend completely, use `"none"`:

```
p19 <- p0 +
  theme(legend.position = "none")
```

Alternatively, we can use relative coordinates (0–1) to give the legend a relative x-y location (Figure 5.11):

```
p20 <- p0 +
  theme(legend.position    = c(1,0), #bottom-right corner
        legend.justification = c(1,0))
```

```
p19 + labs(tag = "p19") + p20 + labs(tag = "p20")
```

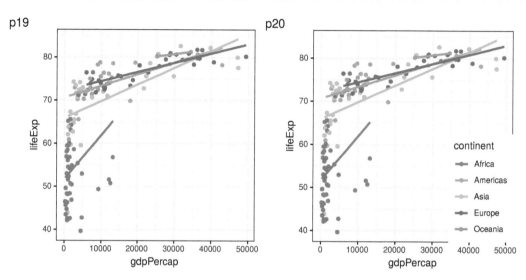

FIGURE 5.11: p19: Setting `theme(legend.position = "none")` removes it. p20: Relative coordinates such as `theme(legend.position = c(1,0)` can by used to place the legend within the plot area.

Further `theme(legend.)` options can be used to change the size, background, spacing, etc., of the legend. However, for modifying the content of the legend, you'll have to use the `guides()` function. Again, `ggplot()`'s defaults are very good, and we rarely need to go into this much tweaking using both the `theme()` and `guides()` functions. But it is good to know what is possible.

For example, this is how to change the number of columns within the legend (Figure 5.12):

```
p21 <- p0 +
  guides(colour = guide_legend(ncol = 2)) +
  theme(legend.position = "top") # moving to the top optional

p21 + labs(tag = "p21")
```

5.6 Saving your plot

In Chapters 12 and 13 we'll show you how to export descriptive text, figures, and tables directly from R to Word/PDF/HTML using the power of R Mark-

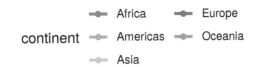

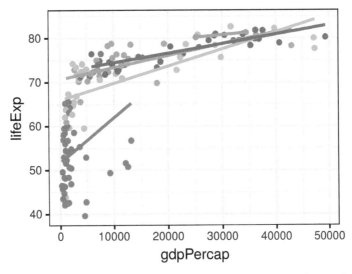

FIGURE 5.12: p21: Changing the number of columns within a legend.

down. The `ggsave()` function, however, can be used to save a single plot into a variety of formats, namely `"pdf"` or `"png"`:

```
ggsave(p0, file = "my_saved_plot.pdf", width = 5, height = 4)
```

If you omit the first argument - the plot object - and call, e.g., `ggsave(file = "plot.png)` it will just save the last plot that got printed.

Text size tip: playing around with the width and height options (they're in inches) can be a convenient way to increase or decrease the relative size of the text on the plot. Look at the relative font sizes of the two versions of the `ggsave()` call, one 5x4, the other one 10x8 (Figure 5.13):

```
ggsave(p0, file = "my_saved_plot_larger.pdf", width = 10, height = 8)
```

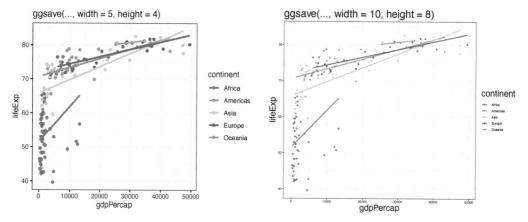

FIGURE 5.13: Experimenting with the width and height options within ggsave() can be used to quickly change how big or small some of the text on your plot looks.

Part II
Data analysis

In the second part of this book, we focus specifically on the business of data analysis, that is, formulating clear questions and seeking to answer them using available datasets.

Again, we emphasise the importance of understanding the underlying data through visualisation, rather than relying on statistical tests or, heaven forbid, the p-value alone.

There are five chapters. Testing for continuous outcome variables (6) leads naturally into linear regression (7). We would expect the majority of actual analysis done by readers to be using the methods in chapter 7 rather than 6. Similarly, testing for categorical outcome variables (8) leads naturally to logistic regression (9), where we would expect the majority of work to focus.

Chapters 6 and 8 however do provide helpful reminders of how to prepare data for these analyses and shouldn't be skipped. time-to-event data (10) introduces survival analysis and includes sections on the manipulation of dates.

6

Working with continuous outcome variables

Continuous data can be measured.
Categorical data can be counted.

6.1 Continuous data

Continuous data is everywhere in healthcare. From physiological measures in patients such as systolic blood pressure or pulmonary function tests, through to population measures like life expectancy or disease incidence, the analysis of continuous outcome measures is common and important.

Our goal in most health data questions, is to draw a conclusion on a comparison between groups. For instance, understanding differences in life expectancy between the year 2002 and 2007 is more useful than simply describing the average life expectancy across all of time.

The basis for comparisons between continuous measures is the *distribution* of the data. That word, as many which have a statistical flavour, brings on the sweats in many people. It needn't. By distribution, we are simply referring to the shape of the data.

6.2 The Question

The examples in this chapter all use the data introduced previously from the amazing Gapminder project[1]. We will start by looking at the life expectancy of populations over time and in different geographical regions.

---

[1] https://www.gapminder.org/

6.3   Get and check the data

```
# Load packages
library(tidyverse)
library(finalfit)
library(gapminder)

# Create object gapdata from object gapminder
gapdata <- gapminder
```

It is vital that datasets be carefully inspected when first read (for help reading data into R see 2.1). The three functions below provide a clear summary, allowing errors or miscoding to be quickly identified. It is particularly important to ensure that any missing data is identified (see Chapter 11). If you don't do this you will regret it! There are many times when an analysis has got to a relatively advanced stage before the researcher was hit by the realisation that the dataset was far from complete.

```
glimpse(gapdata) # each variable as line, variable type, first values
```

```
## Rows: 1,704
## Columns: 6
## $ country   <fct> Afghanistan, Afghanistan, Afghanistan, Afghanistan, Afgha...
## $ continent <fct> Asia, Asia, Asia, Asia, Asia, Asia, Asia, Asia, Asia, Asi...
## $ year      <int> 1952, 1957, 1962, 1967, 1972, 1977, 1982, 1987, 1992, 199...
## $ lifeExp   <dbl> 28.801, 30.332, 31.997, 34.020, 36.088, 38.438, 39.854, 4...
## $ pop       <int> 8425333, 9240934, 10267083, 11537966, 13079460, 14880372,...
## $ gdpPercap <dbl> 779.4453, 820.8530, 853.1007, 836.1971, 739.9811, 786.113...
```

```
missing_glimpse(gapdata) # missing data for each variable
```

```
##                    label var_type     n missing_n missing_percent
## country          country    <fct>  1704         0             0.0
## continent      continent    <fct>  1704         0             0.0
## year                year    <int>  1704         0             0.0
## lifeExp          lifeExp    <dbl>  1704         0             0.0
## pop                  pop    <int>  1704         0             0.0
## gdpPercap      gdpPercap    <dbl>  1704         0             0.0
```

```
ff_glimpse(gapdata) # summary statistics for each variable
```

As can be seen, there are 6 variables, 4 are continuous and 2 are categorical. The categorical variables are already identified as `factors`. There are no missing data. Note that by default, the maximum number of factor levels shown is give,

TABLE 6.1: Gapminder dataset, ff_glimpse: continuous.

label	var_type	n	missing_n	mean	sd	median
year	\<int\>	1704	0	1979.5	17.3	1979.5
lifeExp	\<dbl\>	1704	0	59.5	12.9	60.7
pop	\<int\>	1704	0	29601212.3	106157896.7	7023595.5
gdpPercap	\<dbl\>	1704	0	7215.3	9857.5	3531.8

TABLE 6.2: Gapminder dataset, ff_glimpse: categorical.

label	var_type	n	missing_n	levels_n	levels	levels_count
country	\<fct\>	1704	0	142	-	-
continent	\<fct\>	1704	0	5	"Africa", "Americas", "Asia", "Europe", "Oceania"	624, 300, 396, 360, 24

which is why 142 country names are not printed. This can be adjusted using
`ff_glimpse(gapdata, levels_cut = 142)`

6.4 Plot the data

We will start by comparing life expectancy between the 5 continents of the world in two different years. Always plot your data first. Never skip this step! We are particularly interested in the distribution. There's that word again. The shape of the data. Is it normal? Is it skewed? Does it differ between regions and years?

There are three useful plots which can help here:

- Histograms: examine shape of data and compare groups;
- Q-Q plots: are data normally distributed?
- Box-plots: identify outliers, compare shape and groups.

6.4.1 Histogram

```
gapdata %>%
  filter(year %in% c(2002, 2007)) %>%
  ggplot(aes(x = lifeExp)) +        # remember aes()
  geom_histogram(bins = 20) +       # histogram with 20 bars
  facet_grid(year ~ continent)      # optional: add scales="free"
```

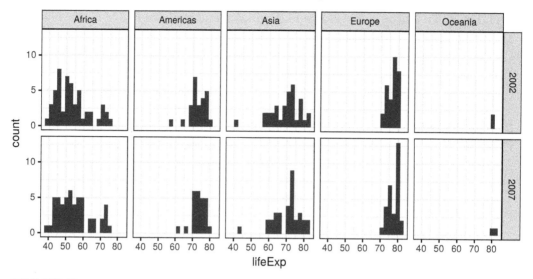

FIGURE 6.1: Histogram: Country life expectancy by continent and year.

What can we see? That life expectancy in Africa is lower than in other regions. That we have little data for Oceania given there are only two countries included, Australia and New Zealand. That Africa and Asia have greater variability in life expectancy by country than in the Americas or Europe. That the data follow a reasonably normal shape, with Africa 2002 a little right skewed.

6.4.2 Quantile-quantile (Q-Q) plot

Quantile-quantile sounds more complicated than it really is. It is a graphical method for comparing the distribution (think shape) of our own data to a theoretical distribution, such as the normal distribution. In this context, quantiles are just cut points which divide our data into bins each containing the same number of observations. For example, if we have the life expectancy for 100 countries, then quartiles (note the quar-) for life expectancy are the three ages which split the observations into 4 groups each containing 25 countries. A Q-Q plot simply plots the quantiles for our data against the theoretical quantiles for a particular distribution (the default shown below is the normal distribution). If our data follow that distribution (e.g., normal), then our data points fall on the theoretical straight line.

```
gapdata %>%
  filter(year %in% c(2002, 2007)) %>%
  ggplot(aes(sample = lifeExp)) +      # Q-Q plot requires 'sample'
  geom_qq() +                          # defaults to normal distribution
  geom_qq_line(colour = "blue") +      # add the theoretical line
  facet_grid(year ~ continent)
```

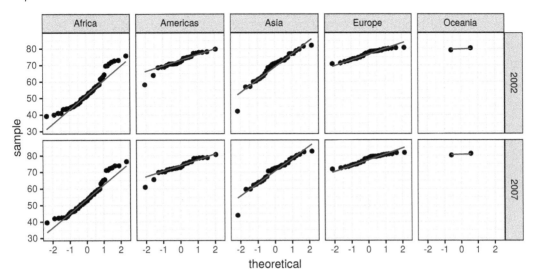

FIGURE 6.2: Q-Q plot: Country life expectancy by continent and year.

What can we see? We are looking to see if the data (dots) follow the straight line which we included in the plot. These do reasonably, except for Africa which is curved upwards at each end. This is the right skew we could see on the histograms too. If your data do not follow a normal distribution, then you should avoid using a *t*-test or ANOVA when comparing groups. Non-parametric tests are one alternative and are described in Section 6.9.

We are frequently asked about the pros and cons of checking for normality using a statistical test, such as the Shapiro-Wilk normality test. We don't recommend it. The test is often non-significant when the number of observations is small but the data look skewed, and often significant when the number of observations is high but the data look reasonably normal on inspection of plots. It is therefore not useful in practice - common sense should prevail.

6.4.3 Boxplot

Boxplots are our preferred method for comparing a continuous variable such as life expectancy across a categorical explanatory variable. For continuous data, box plots are a lot more appropriate than bar plots with error bars (also known as dynamite plots). We intentionally do not even show you how to make dynamite plots.

The box represents the median (bold horizontal line in the middle) and interquartile range (where 50% of the data sits). The lines (whiskers) extend to the lowest and highest values that are still within 1.5 times the interquartile range. Outliers (anything outwith the whiskers) are represented as points.

The beautiful boxplot thus contains information not only on central tendency (median), but on the variation in the data and the distribution of the data, for instance a skew should be obvious.

```
gapdata %>%
  filter(year %in% c(2002, 2007)) %>%
  ggplot(aes(x = continent, y = lifeExp)) +
  geom_boxplot() +
  facet_wrap(~ year)
```

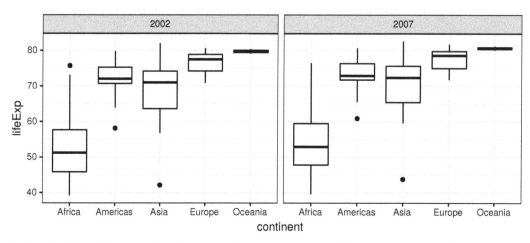

FIGURE 6.3: Boxplot: Country life expectancy by continent and year.

What can we see? The median life expectancy is lower in Africa than in any other continent. The variation in life expectancy is greatest in Africa and smallest in Oceania. The data in Africa looks skewed, particularly in 2002 - the lines/whiskers are unequal lengths.

We can add further arguments to adjust the plot to our liking. We particularly encourage the inclusion of the actual data points, here using `geom_jitter()`.

```
gapdata %>%
  filter(year %in% c(2002, 2007)) %>%
  ggplot(aes(x = factor(year), y = lifeExp)) +
  geom_boxplot(aes(fill = continent)) +      # add colour to boxplots
  geom_jitter(alpha = 0.4) +                 # alpha = transparency
  facet_wrap(~ continent, ncol = 5) +        # spread by continent
  theme(legend.position = "none") +          # remove legend
  xlab("Year") +                             # label x-axis
  ylab("Life expectancy (years)") +          # label y-axis
  ggtitle(
    "Life expectancy by continent in 2002 v 2007") # add title
```

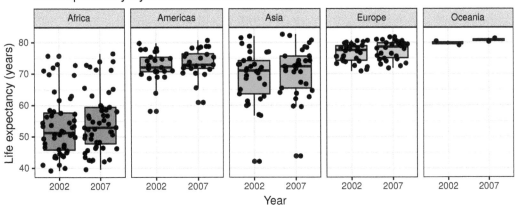

FIGURE 6.4: Boxplot with jitter points: Country life expectancy by continent and year.

6.5 Compare the means of two groups

6.5.1 *t*-test

A *t*-test is used to compare the means of two groups of continuous measurements. Volumes have been written about this elsewhere, and we won't rehearse it here.

There are a few variations of the *t*-test. We will use two here. The most useful in our context is a two-sample test of independent groups. Repeated-measures data, such as comparing the same countries in different years, can be analysed using a paired *t*-test.

6.5.2 Two-sample *t*-tests

Referring to Figure 6.3, let's compare life expectancy between Asia and Europe for 2007. What is imperative is that you decide what sort of difference exists by looking at the boxplot, rather than relying on the *t*-test output. The median for Europe is clearly higher than in Asia. The distributions overlap, but it looks likely that Europe has a higher life expectancy than Asia.

By running the two-sample *t*-test here, we make the assumption that life expectancy in each country represents an independent measurement of life expectancy in the continent as a whole. This isn't quite right if you think about it carefully.

Imagine a room full of enthusiastic geniuses learning R. They arrived today from various parts of the country. For reasons known only to you, you want to know whether the average (mean) height of those wearing glasses is different to those with perfect vision.

You measure the height of each person in the room, check them for glasses, and run a two-sample *t*-test.

In statistical terms, your room represents a sample from an underlying population. Your ability to answer the question accurately relies on a number of factors. For instance, how many people are in the room? The more there are, the more certain you can be about the mean measurement in your groups being close to the mean measurement in the overall population.

What is also crucial is that your room is a representative sample of the population. Are the observations independent, i.e., is each observation unrelated to the others?

If you have inadvertently included a family of bespectacled nerdy giants, not typical of those in the country as a whole, your estimate will be wrong and your conclusion incorrect.

So in our example of countries and continents, you have to assume that the mean life expectancy of each country does not depend on the life expectancies of other countries in the group. In other words, that each measurement is independent.

```
ttest_data <- gapdata %>%                          # save as object ttest_data
  filter(year == 2007) %>%                         # 2007 only
  filter(continent %in% c("Asia", "Europe"))       # Asia/Europe only

ttest_result <- ttest_data %>%                     # example using pipe
  t.test(lifeExp ~ continent, data = .)            # note data = ., see below
ttest_result
```

```
##
##  Welch Two Sample t-test
##
## data:  lifeExp by continent
## t = -4.6468, df = 41.529, p-value = 3.389e-05
## alternative hypothesis: true difference in means is not equal to 0
## 95 percent confidence interval:
##   -9.926525 -3.913705
## sample estimates:
##    mean in group Asia mean in group Europe
##             70.72848             77.64860
```

The Welch two-sample *t*-test is the most flexible and copes with differences in variance (variability) between groups, as in this example. The difference in means is provided at the bottom of the output. The *t*-value, degrees of freedom (df) and *p*-value are all provided. The *p*-value is 0.00003.

We used the assignment arrow to save the results of the *t*-test into a new object called `ttest_result`. If you look at the Environment tab, you should see `ttest_result` there. If you click on it - to view it - you'll realise that it's not structured like a table, but a list of different pieces of information. The structure of the *t*-test object is shown in Figure 6.5.

Name	Type	Value
⊙ ttest_result	list [10] (S3: htest)	List of length 10
◉ statistic	double [1]	−4.646757
◉ parameter	double [1]	41.52851
p.value	double [1]	3.38922e-05
conf.int	double [2]	−9.93 −3.91
◉ estimate	double [2]	70.7 77.6
◉ null.value	double [1]	0
stderr	double [1]	1.489235
alternative	character [1]	'two.sided'
method	character [1]	'Welch Two Sample t-test'
data.name	character [1]	'lifeExp by continent'

FIGURE 6.5: A list object that is the result of a t-test in R. We will show you ways to access these numbers and how to wrangle them into more familiar tables/tibbles.

The *p*-value, for instance, can be accessed like this:

```
ttest_result$p.value # Extracted element of result object
```

```
## [1] 3.38922e-05
```

The confidence interval of the difference in mean life expectancy between the two continents:

```
ttest_result$conf.int # Extracted element of result object
```

```
## [1] -9.926525 -3.913705
## attr(,"conf.level")
## [1] 0.95
```

The **broom** package provides useful methods for 'tidying' common model

TABLE 6.3: Results of a t-test wrangled into a table using library(broom).

estimate	estimate1	estimate2	statistic	p.value	parameter	conf.low	conf.high
-6.920115	70.72848	77.6486	-4.646757	3.39e-05	41.52851	-9.926525	-3.913705

outputs into a `tibble`. So instead of accessing the various bits of information by checking the `names()` and then using the `$` operator, we can use functions called `tidy()` and `glance()` to wrangle the statistical output into a table:

**Reminder: When the pipe sends data to the wrong place: use `data =`
. to redirect it**

In the code above, the `data = .` bit is necessary because the pipe usually sends data to the beginning of function brackets. So `gapdata %>% t.test(lifeExp ~ continent)` would be equivalent to `t.test(gapdata, lifeExp ~ continent)`. However, this is not an order that `t.test()` will accept. `t.test()` wants us to specify the formula first, and then wants the data these variables are present in. So we have to use the `.` to tell the pipe to send the data to the second argument of `t.test()`, not the first.

6.5.3 Paired *t*-tests

Consider that we want to compare the difference in life expectancy in Asian countries between 2002 and 2007. The overall difference is not impressive in the boxplot.

We can plot differences at the country level directly.

```
paired_data <- gapdata %>%              # save as object paired_data
  filter(year %in% c(2002, 2007)) %>%   # 2002 and 2007 only
  filter(continent == "Asia")           # Asia only

paired_data %>%
  ggplot(aes(x = year, y = lifeExp,
             group = country)) +        # for individual country lines
  geom_line()
```

What is the difference in life expectancy for each individual country? We don't usually have to produce this directly, but here is one method.

```
paired_table <- paired_data %>%           # save object paired_data
  select(country, year, lifeExp) %>%      # select vars interest
  pivot_wider(names_from = year,          # put years in columns
              values_from = lifeExp) %>%
  mutate(
    dlifeExp = `2007` - `2002`            # difference in means
```

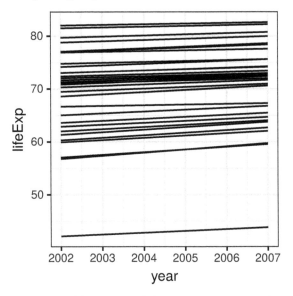

FIGURE 6.6: Line plot: Change in life expectancy in Asian countries from 2002 to 2007.

```
  )
paired_table
```

```
## # A tibble: 33 x 4
##    country          `2002` `2007` dlifeExp
##    <fct>             <dbl>  <dbl>    <dbl>
##  1 Afghanistan        42.1   43.8     1.70
##  2 Bahrain            74.8   75.6     0.84
##  3 Bangladesh         62.0   64.1     2.05
##  4 Cambodia           56.8   59.7     2.97
##  5 China              72.0   73.0    0.933
##  6 Hong Kong, China   81.5   82.2    0.713
##  7 India              62.9   64.7     1.82
##  8 Indonesia          68.6   70.6     2.06
##  9 Iran               69.5   71.0     1.51
## 10 Iraq               57.0   59.5     2.50
## # ... with 23 more rows
```

```
# Mean of difference in years
paired_table %>% summarise( mean(dlifeExp) )
```

```
## # A tibble: 1 x 1
##    `mean(dlifeExp)`
##              <dbl>
## 1             1.49
```

On average, therefore, there is an increase in life expectancy of 1.5 years in Asian countries between 2002 and 2007. Let's test whether this number differs from zero with a paired *t*-test:

```
paired_data %>%
  t.test(lifeExp ~ year, data = ., paired = TRUE)
```

```
##
##  Paired t-test
##
## data:  lifeExp by year
## t = -14.338, df = 32, p-value = 1.758e-15
## alternative hypothesis: true difference in means is not equal to 0
## 95 percent confidence interval:
##  -1.706941 -1.282271
## sample estimates:
## mean of the differences
##               -1.494606
```

The results show a highly significant difference (p-value $= 0.000000000000002$).
The average difference of 1.5 years is highly consistent between countries, as
shown on the line plot, and this differs from zero. It is up to you the investigator to interpret the relevance of the effect size of 1.5 years in reporting
the finding. A highly significant p-value does not necessarily mean there is a
(clinically) significant change between the two groups (or in this example, two
time points).

6.5.4   What if I run the wrong test?

As an exercise, we can repeat this analysis comparing these data in an unpaired manner. The resulting (unpaired) p-value is 0.460. Remember, a paired
t-test of the same data (life expectancies of Asian countries in 2002 and 2007)
showed a very different, significant result. In this case, running an unpaired
two-sample t-test is just wrong - as the data are indeed paired. It is important that the investigator really understands the data and the underlying
processes/relationships within it. R will not know and therefore cannot warn
you if you run the wrong test.

6.6   Compare the mean of one group: one sample t-tests

We can use a t-test to determine whether the mean of a distribution is different
to a specific value. For instance, we can test whether the mean life expectancy
in each continent was significantly different from 77 years in 2007. We have
included some extra code here to demonstrate how to run multiple tests in
one pipe function.

```
gapdata %>%
  filter(year == 2007) %>%          # 2007 only
  group_by(continent) %>%           # split by continent
  do(                               # dplyr function
    t.test(.$lifeExp, mu = 77) %>%  # compare mean to 77 years
      tidy()                        # tidy into tibble
  )
```

```
## # A tibble: 5 x 9
## # Groups:   continent [5]
##   continent estimate statistic  p.value parameter conf.low conf.high method
##   <fct>        <dbl>     <dbl>    <dbl>     <dbl>    <dbl>     <dbl> <chr>
## 1 Africa        54.8    -16.6  3.15e-22        51     52.1      57.5 One S~
## 2 Americas      73.6     -3.82 8.32e- 4        24     71.8      75.4 One S~
## 3 Asia          70.7     -4.52 7.88e- 5        32     67.9      73.6 One S~
## 4 Europe        77.6      1.19 2.43e- 1        29     76.5      78.8 One S~
## 5 Oceania       80.7      7.22 8.77e- 2         1     74.2      87.3 One S~
## # ... with 1 more variable: alternative <chr>
```

The mean life expectancy for Europe and Oceania do not significantly differ from 77, while the others do. In particular, look at the confidence intervals of the results above (conf.low and conf.high columns) and whether they include or exclude 77. For instance, Oceania's confidence intervals are especially wide as the dataset only includes two countries. Therefore, we can't conclude that its value isn't different to 77, but that we don't have enough observations and the estimate is uncertain. It doesn't make sense to report the results of a statistical test - whether the *p*-value is significant or not - without assessing the confidence intervals.

6.6.1 Interchangeability of *t*-tests

Furthermore, remember how we calculated the table of differences in the paired *t*-test section? We can use these differences for each pair of observations (country's life expectancy in 2002 and 2007) to run a simple one-sample *t*-test instead:

```
# note that we're using dlifeExp
# so the differences we calculated above
t.test(paired_table$dlifeExp, mu = 0)
```

```
##
##  One Sample t-test
##
## data:  paired_table$dlifeExp
## t = 14.338, df = 32, p-value = 1.758e-15
## alternative hypothesis: true mean is not equal to 0
## 95 percent confidence interval:
##   1.282271 1.706941
## sample estimates:
## mean of x
```

```
##   1.494606
```

Notice how this result is identical to the paired *t*-test.

6.7   Compare the means of more than two groups

It may be that our question is set around a hypothesis involving more than two groups. For example, we may be interested in comparing life expectancy across 3 continents such as the Americas, Europe and Asia.

6.7.1   Plot the data

```
gapdata %>%
  filter(year == 2007) %>%
  filter(continent %in%
          c("Americas", "Europe", "Asia")) %>%
  ggplot(aes(x = continent, y=lifeExp)) +
  geom_boxplot()
```

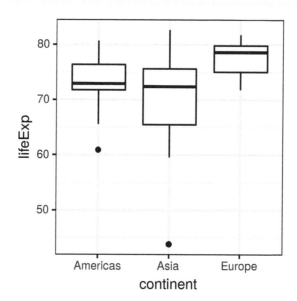

FIGURE 6.7: Boxplot: Life expectancy in selected continents for 2007.

6.7.2   ANOVA

Analysis of variance is a collection of statistical tests which can be used to test the difference in means between two or more groups.

In base R form, it produces an ANOVA table which includes an F-test. This
so-called omnibus test tells you whether there are any differences in the comparison of means of the included groups. Again, it is important to plot carefully
and be clear what question you are asking.

```
aov_data <- gapdata %>%
  filter(year == 2007) %>%
  filter(continent %in% c("Americas", "Europe", "Asia"))

fit = aov(lifeExp ~ continent, data = aov_data)
summary(fit)
```

```
##             Df Sum Sq Mean Sq F value   Pr(>F)
## continent    2  755.6   377.8   11.63 3.42e-05 ***
## Residuals   85 2760.3    32.5
## ---
## Signif. codes:  0 '***' 0.001 '**' 0.01 '*' 0.05 '.' 0.1 ' ' 1
```

We can conclude from the significant F-test that the mean life expectancy
across the three continents is not the same. This does not mean that all included groups are significantly different from each other. As above, the output
can be neatened up using the tidy function.

```
library(broom)
gapdata %>%
  filter(year == 2007) %>%
  filter(continent %in% c("Americas", "Europe", "Asia")) %>%
  aov(lifeExp~continent, data = .) %>%
  tidy()
```

```
## # A tibble: 2 x 6
##   term          df sumsq meansq statistic   p.value
##   <chr>      <dbl> <dbl>  <dbl>     <dbl>     <dbl>
## 1 continent      2  756.   378.      11.6 0.0000342
## 2 Residuals     85 2760.   32.5       NA        NA
```

6.7.3 Assumptions

As with the normality assumption of the t-test (for example, Sections 6.4.1
and 6.4.2), there are assumptions of the ANOVA model. These assumptions
are shared with linear regression and are covered in the next chapter, as linear
regression lends itself to illustrate and explain these concepts well. Suffice
to say that diagnostic plots can be produced to check that the assumptions
are fulfilled. library(ggfortify) includes a function called autoplot() that can be
used to quickly create diagnostic plots, including the Q-Q plot that we showed
before:

```
library(ggfortify)
autoplot(fit)
```

```
## Warning: `arrange_()` is deprecated as of dplyr 0.7.0.
## Please use `arrange()` instead.
## See vignette('programming') for more help
## This warning is displayed once every 8 hours.
## Call `lifecycle::last_warnings()` to see where this warning was generated.
```

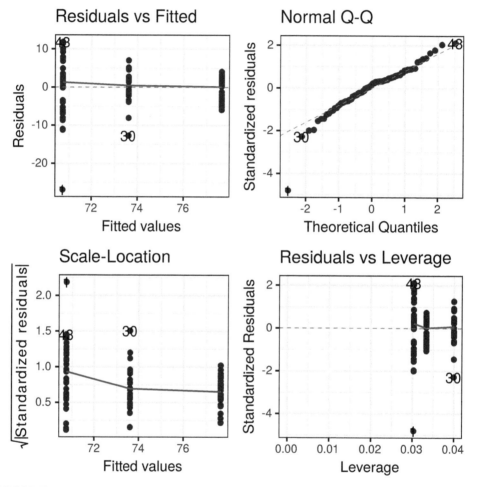

FIGURE 6.8: Diagnostic plots: ANOVA model of life expectancy by continent for 2007.

6.8 Multiple testing

6.8.1 Pairwise testing and multiple comparisons

When the F-test is significant, we will often want to determine where the differences lie. This should of course be obvious from the boxplot you have made. However, some are fixated on the *p*-value!

```
pairwise.t.test(aov_data$lifeExp, aov_data$continent,
                p.adjust.method = "bonferroni")
```

```
##
##  Pairwise comparisons using t tests with pooled SD
##
## data:  aov_data$lifeExp and aov_data$continent
##
##        Americas Asia
## Asia   0.180    -
## Europe 0.031    1.9e-05
##
## P value adjustment method: bonferroni
```

A matrix of pairwise *p*-values can be produced using the code above. Here we can see that there is good evidence of a difference in means between Europe and Asia.

We have to keep in mind that the *p*-value's significance level of 0.05 means we have a 5% chance of finding a difference in our samples which doesn't exist in the overall population.

Therefore, the more statistical tests performed, the greater the chances of a false positive result. This is also known as type I error - finding a difference when no difference exists.

There are three approaches to dealing with situations where multiple statistical tests are performed. The first is not to perform any correction at all. Some advocate that the best approach is simply to present the results of all the tests that were performed, and let sceptical readers make adjustments for themselves. This is attractive, but presupposes a sophisticated readership who will take the time to consider the results in their entirety.

The second and classical approach is to control for the so-called family-wise error rate. The "Bonferroni" correction is the most famous and most conservative, where the threshold for significance is lowered in proportion to the number of comparisons made. For example, if three comparisons are made, the threshold for significance should be lowered to 0.017. Equivalently, all *p*-values should be multiplied by the number of tests performed (in this case 3).

The adjusted values can then be compared to a threshold of 0.05, as is the case above. The Bonferroni method is particularly conservative, meaning that type II errors may occur (failure to identify true differences, or false negatives) in favour or minimising type I errors (false positives).

The third approach controls for something called false-discovery rate. The development of these methods has been driven in part by the needs of areas of science where many different statistical tests are performed at the same time, for instance, examining the influence of 1000 genes simultaneously. In these hypothesis-generating settings, a higher tolerance to type I errors may be preferable to missing potential findings through type II errors. You can see in our example, that the *p*-values are lower with the `fdr` correction than the `Bonferroni` correction ones.

```
pairwise.t.test(aov_data$lifeExp, aov_data$continent,
                p.adjust.method = "fdr")
```

```
##
##   Pairwise comparisons using t tests with pooled SD
##
## data:   aov_data$lifeExp and aov_data$continent
##
##        Americas Asia
## Asia   0.060    -
## Europe 0.016    1.9e-05
##
## P value adjustment method: fdr
```

Try not to get too hung up on this. Be sensible. Plot the data and look for differences. Focus on effect size. For instance, what is the actual difference in life expectancy in years, rather than the *p*-value of a comparison test. Choose a method which fits with your overall aims. If you are generating hypotheses which you will proceed to test with other methods, the `fdr` approach may be preferable. If you are trying to capture robust effects and want to minimise type II errors, use a family-wise approach.

If your head is spinning at this point, don't worry. The rest of the book will continuously revisit these and other similar concepts, e.g., "know your data", "be sensible, look at the effect size", using several different examples and datasets. So do not feel like you should be able to understand everything immediately. Furthermore, these things are easier to conceptualise when using your own dataset - especially if that's something you've put your blood, sweat and tears into collecting.

6.9 Non-parametric tests

What if your data is a different shape to normal, or the ANOVA assumptions are not fulfilled (see linear regression chapter)? As always, be sensible and think what drives your measurements in the first place. Would your data be expected to be normally distributed given the data-generating process?

For instance, if you are examining length of hospital stay it is likely that your data are highly right skewed - most patients are discharged from hospital in a few days while a smaller number stay for a long time. Is a comparison of means ever going to be the correct approach here? Perhaps you should consider a time-to-event analysis for instance (see Chapter 10).

If a comparison of means approach is reasonable, but the normality assumption is not fulfilled there are two approaches,

1. Transform the data;
2. Perform non-parametric tests.

6.9.1 Transforming data

Remember, the Welch *t*-test is reasonably robust to divergence from the normality assumption, so small deviations can be safely ignored.

Otherwise, the data can be transformed to another scale to deal with a skew. A natural `log` scale is common.

TABLE 6.4: Transformations that can be applied to skewed data. For left skewed data, subtract all values from a constant greater than the maximum value.

Distribution	Transformation	Function
Moderate right skew (+)	Square-root	sqrt()
Substantial right skew (++)	Natural log*	log()
Substantial right skew (+++)	Base-10 log*	log10()

Note:
If data contain zero values, add a small constant to all values.

```
africa2002 <- gapdata %>%        # save as africa2002
  filter(year == 2002) %>%       # only 2002
  filter(continent == "Africa") %>%   # only Africa
  select(country, lifeExp) %>%   # only these variables
  mutate(
```

```
    lifeExp_log = log(lifeExp)              # log life expectancy
  )
head(africa2002)                           # inspect
```

```
## # A tibble: 6 x 3
##    country       lifeExp lifeExp_log
##    <fct>           <dbl>       <dbl>
## 1 Algeria          71.0        4.26
## 2 Angola           41.0        3.71
## 3 Benin            54.4        4.00
## 4 Botswana         46.6        3.84
## 5 Burkina Faso     50.6        3.92
## 6 Burundi          47.4        3.86
```

```
africa2002 %>%
  # pivot lifeExp and lifeExp_log values to same column (for easy plotting):
  pivot_longer(contains("lifeExp")) %>%
  ggplot(aes(x = value)) +
  geom_histogram(bins = 15) +            # make histogram
  facet_wrap(~name, scales = "free")     # facet with axes free to vary
```

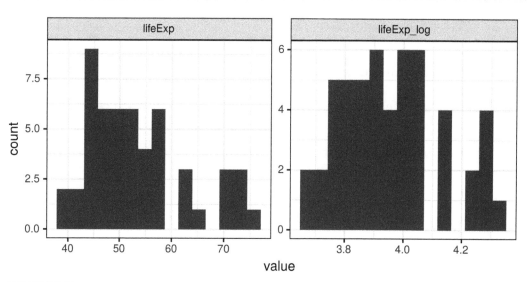

FIGURE 6.9: Histogram: Log transformation of life expectancy for countries in Africa 2002.

This has worked well here. The right skew on the Africa data has been dealt with by the transformation. A parametric test such as a *t*-test can now be performed.

6.9.2   Non-parametric test for comparing two groups

The Mann-Whitney U test is also called the Wilcoxon rank-sum test and uses a rank-based method to compare two groups (note the Wilcoxon signed-rank test is for paired data). Rank-based just means ordering your grouped continuous data from smallest to largest value and assigning a rank (1, 2, 3 ...) to each measurement.

We can use it to test for a difference in life expectancies for African countries between 1982 and 2007. Let's do a histogram, Q-Q plot and boxplot first.

```r
africa_data <- gapdata %>%
  filter(year %in% c(1982, 2007)) %>%     # only 1982 and 2007
  filter(continent %in% c("Africa"))      # only Africa

p1 <- africa_data %>%                     # save plot as p1
  ggplot(aes(x = lifeExp)) +
  geom_histogram(bins = 15) +
  facet_wrap(~year)

p2 <- africa_data %>%                     # save plot as p2
  ggplot(aes(sample = lifeExp)) +         # `sample` for Q-Q plot
  geom_qq() +
  geom_qq_line(colour = "blue") +
  facet_wrap(~year)

p3 <- africa_data %>%                     # save plot as p3
  ggplot(aes(x = factor(year),            # try without factor(year) to
             y = lifeExp)) +              # see the difference
  geom_boxplot(aes(fill = factor(year))) + # colour boxplot
  geom_jitter(alpha = 0.4) +              # add data points
  theme(legend.position = "none")         # remove legend

library(patchwork)                        # great for combining plots
p1 / p2 | p3
```

The data is a little skewed based on the histograms and Q-Q plots. The difference between 1982 and 2007 is not particularly striking on the boxplot.

```r
africa_data %>%
  wilcox.test(lifeExp ~ year, data = .)
```

```
##
##  Wilcoxon rank sum test with continuity correction
##
## data:  lifeExp by year
## W = 1130, p-value = 0.1499
## alternative hypothesis: true location shift is not equal to 0
```

6.9.3   Non-parametric test for comparing more than two groups

The non-parametric equivalent to ANOVA, is the Kruskal-Wallis test. It can be used in base R, or via the **finalfit** package below.

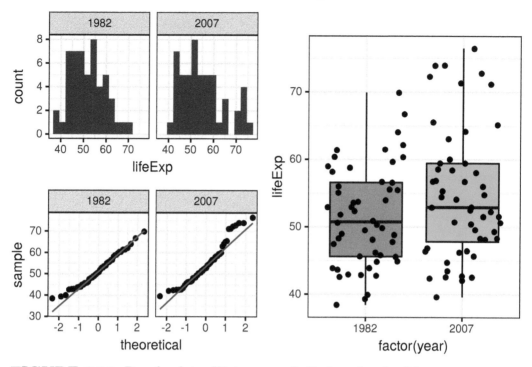

FIGURE 6.10: Panels plots: Histogram, Q-Q, boxplot for life expectancy in Africa 1992 v 2007.

```
library(broom)
gapdata %>%
  filter(year == 2007) %>%
  filter(continent %in% c("Americas", "Europe", "Asia")) %>%
  kruskal.test(lifeExp~continent, data = .) %>%
  tidy()
```

```
## # A tibble: 1 x 4
##   statistic  p.value parameter method
##       <dbl>    <dbl>     <int> <chr>
## 1      21.6 0.0000202         2 Kruskal-Wallis rank sum test
```

6.10   Finalfit approach

The **finalfit** package provides an easy to use interface for performing non-parametric hypothesis tests. Any number of explanatory variables can be tested against a so-called dependent variable. In this case, this is equivalent to a typical Table 1 in healthcare study.

```
dependent <- "year"
explanatory <- c("lifeExp", "pop", "gdpPercap")
africa_data %>%
  mutate(
    year = factor(year)
  ) %>%
  summary_factorlist(dependent, explanatory,
                     cont = "median", p = TRUE)
```

Note that the *p*-values above have not been corrected for multiple testing.

TABLE 6.5: Life expectancy, population and GDPperCap in Africa 1982 vs 2007.

label	levels	1982	2007	p
lifeExp	Median (IQR)	50.8 (11.0)	52.9 (11.6)	0.149
pop	Median (IQR)	5668228.5 (8218654.0)	10093310.5 (16454428.0)	0.033
gdpPercap	Median (IQR)	1323.7 (1958.9)	1452.3 (3130.6)	0.503

There are many other options available for this function which are covered throughout this book. For instance, If you wish to consider only some variables as non-parametric and summarise with a median, then this can be specified using

```
dependent <- "year"
explanatory <- c("lifeExp", "pop", "gdpPercap")
africa_data %>%
  mutate(
    year = factor(year)
  ) %>%
  summary_factorlist(dependent, explanatory,
                     cont_nonpara =  c(1, 3),            # variable 1&3 are non-parametric
                     cont_range = TRUE,                  # lower and upper quartile
                     p = TRUE,                           # include hypothesis test
                     p_cont_para = "t.test",             # use t.test/aov for parametric
                     add_row_totals = TRUE,              # row totals
                     include_row_missing_col = FALSE,    # missing values row totals
                     add_dependent_label = TRUE)         # dependent label
```

TABLE 6.6: Life expectancy, population and GDPperCap in Africa 1982 vs 2007.

Dependent: year	Total N		1982	2007	p
lifeExp	104	Median (IQR)	50.8 (45.6 to 56.6)	52.9 (47.8 to 59.4)	0.149
pop	104	Mean (SD)	9602857.4 (13456243.4)	17875763.3 (24917726.2)	0.038
gdpPercap	104	Median (IQR)	1323.7 (828.7 to 2787.6)	1452.3 (863.0 to 3993.5)	0.503

6.11   Conclusions

Continuous data is frequently encountered in a healthcare setting. Liberal use of plotting is required to really understand the underlying data. Comparisons can be easily made between two or more groups of data, but always remember what you are actually trying to analyse and don't become fixated on the p-value. In the next chapter, we will explore the comparison of two continuous variables together with multivariable models of datasets.

6.12   Exercises

6.12.1   Exercise

Make a histogram, Q-Q plot, and a box-plot for the life expectancy for a continent of your choice, but for all years. Do the data appear normally distributed?

6.12.2   Exercise

1. Select any 2 years in any continent and perform a t-test to determine whether mean life expectancy is significantly different. Remember to plot your data first.

2. Extract only the p-value from your t.test() output.

6.12.3   Exercise

In 2007, in which continents did mean life expectancy differ from 70?

6.12.4   Exercise

1. Use ANOVA to determine if the population changed significantly through the 1990s/2000s in individual continents.

6.13   Solutions

Solution to Exercise 6.12.1:

```
## Make a histogram, Q-Q plot, and a box-plot for the life expectancy
## for a continent of your choice, but for all years.
## Do the data appear normally distributed?

asia_data <- gapdata %>%
  filter(continent %in% c("Asia"))

p1 <- asia_data %>%
  ggplot(aes(x = lifeExp)) +
  geom_histogram(bins = 15)

p2 <- asia_data %>%
  ggplot(aes(sample = lifeExp)) +              # sample =  for Q-Q plot
  geom_qq() +
  geom_qq_line(colour = "blue")

p3 <- asia_data %>%
  ggplot(aes(x = year, y = lifeExp)) +
  geom_boxplot(aes(fill = factor(year))) +  # optional: year as factor
  geom_jitter(alpha = 0.4) +
  theme(legend.position = "none")

library(patchwork)
p1 / p2 | p3
```

Solution to Exercise 6.12.2:

```
## Select any 2 years in any continent and perform a *t*-test to
## determine whether mean life expectancy is significantly different.
## Remember to plot your data first.

asia_2years <- asia_data %>%
  filter(year %in% c(1952, 1972))

p1 <- asia_2years %>%
  ggplot(aes(x = lifeExp)) +
  geom_histogram(bins = 15) +
  facet_wrap(~year)

p2 <- asia_2years %>%
  ggplot(aes(sample = lifeExp)) +
  geom_qq() +
  geom_qq_line(colour = "blue") +
  facet_wrap(~year)

p3 <- asia_2years %>%
  ggplot(aes(x = factor(year), y = lifeExp)) +
  geom_boxplot(aes(fill = factor(year))) +
  geom_jitter(alpha = 0.4) +
  theme(legend.position = "none")

library(patchwork)
p1 / p2 | p3
```

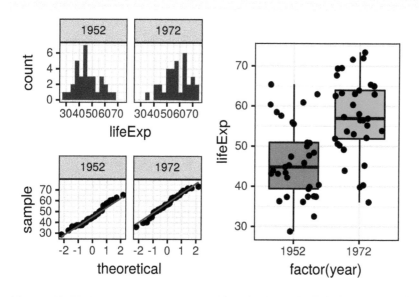

```
asia_2years %>%
  t.test(lifeExp ~ year, data = .)
```

```
##
##  Welch Two Sample t-test
##
## data:  lifeExp by year
## t = -4.7007, df = 63.869, p-value = 1.428e-05
## alternative hypothesis: true difference in means is not equal to 0
```

```
## 95 percent confidence interval:
##  -15.681981  -6.327769
## sample estimates:
## mean in group 1952 mean in group 1972
##           46.31439           57.31927
```

Solution to Exercise 6.12.3:

```
## In 2007, in which continents did mean life expectancy differ from 70
gapdata %>%
  filter(year == 2007) %>%
  group_by(continent) %>%
  do(
    t.test(.$lifeExp, mu = 70) %>%
      tidy()
  )
```

```
## # A tibble: 5 x 9
## # Groups:   continent [5]
##   continent estimate statistic  p.value parameter conf.low conf.high method
##   <fct>        <dbl>     <dbl>    <dbl>     <dbl>    <dbl>     <dbl> <chr>
## 1 Africa        54.8    -11.4  1.33e-15        51     52.1      57.5 One S~
## 2 Americas      73.6      4.06 4.50e- 4        24     71.8      75.4 One S~
## 3 Asia          70.7      0.525 6.03e- 1       32     67.9      73.6 One S~
## 4 Europe        77.6     14.1  1.76e-14        29     76.5      78.8 One S~
## 5 Oceania       80.7     20.8  3.06e- 2         1     74.2      87.3 One S~
## # ... with 1 more variable: alternative <chr>
```

Solution to Exercise 6.12.4:

```
## Use Kruskal-Wallis to determine if the mean population changed
## significantly through the 1990s/2000s in individual continents.

gapdata %>%
  filter(year >= 1990) %>%
  ggplot(aes(x = factor(year), y = pop)) +
  geom_boxplot() +
  facet_wrap(~continent)
```

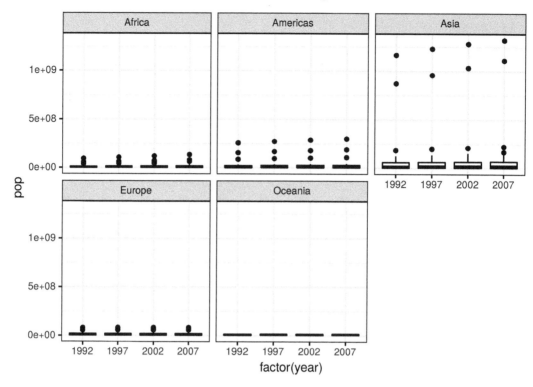

```
gapdata %>%
  filter(year >= 1990) %>%
  group_by(continent) %>%
  do(
    kruskal.test(pop ~ year, data = .) %>%
      tidy()
  )
```

```
## # A tibble: 5 x 5
## # Groups:   continent [5]
##   continent statistic p.value parameter method
##   <fct>         <dbl>   <dbl>     <int> <chr>
## 1 Africa         2.10   0.553         3 Kruskal-Wallis rank sum test
## 2 Americas       0.847  0.838         3 Kruskal-Wallis rank sum test
## 3 Asia           1.57   0.665         3 Kruskal-Wallis rank sum test
## 4 Europe         0.207  0.977         3 Kruskal-Wallis rank sum test
## 5 Oceania        1.67   0.644         3 Kruskal-Wallis rank sum test
```

7

Linear regression

Smoking is one of the leading causes of statistics.
Fletcher Knebel

7.1 Regression

Regression is a method by which we can determine the existence and strength of the relationship between two or more variables. This can be thought of as drawing lines, ideally straight lines, through data points.

Linear regression is our method of choice for examining continuous outcome variables. Broadly, there are often two separate goals in regression:

- Prediction: fitting a predictive model to an observed dataset, then using that model to make predictions about an outcome from a new set of explanatory variables;
- Explanation: fit a model to explain the inter-relationships between a set of variables.

Figure 7.1 unifies the terms we will use throughout. A clear scientific question should define our explanatory variable of interest (x), which sometimes gets called an exposure, predictor, or independent variable. Our outcome of interest will be referred to as the dependent variable or outcome (y); it is sometimes referred to as the response. In simple linear regression, there is a single explanatory variable and a single dependent variable, and we will sometimes refer to this as *univariable linear regression*. When there is more than one explanatory variable, we will call this *multivariable regression*. Avoid the term *multivariate regression*, which means more than one dependent variable. We don't use this method and we suggest you don't either!

Note that in linear regression, the dependent variable is always continuous;

it cannot be a categorical variable. The explanatory variables can be either continuous or categorical.

7.1.1 The Question (1)

We will illustrate our examples of linear regression using a classical question which is important to many of us! This is the relationship between coffee consumption and blood pressure (and therefore cardiovascular events, such as myocardial infarction and stroke). There has been a lot of backwards and forwards over the decades about whether coffee is harmful, has no effect, or is in fact beneficial.

Figure 7.1 shows a linear regression example. Each point is a person. The explanatory variable is average number of cups of coffee per day (x) and systolic blood pressure is the dependent variable (y). This next bit is important! **These data are made up, fake, randomly generated, fabricated, not real.**[1] So please do not alter your coffee habit on the basis of these plots!

7.1.2 Fitting a regression line

Simple linear regression uses the *ordinary least squares* method for fitting. The details are beyond the scope of this book, but if you want to get out the linear algebra/matrix maths you did in high school, an enjoyable afternoon can be spent proving to yourself how it actually works.

Figure 7.2 aims to make this easy to understand. The maths defines a line which best fits the data provided. For the line to fit best, the distances between it and the observed data should be as small as possible. The distance from each observed point to the line is called a *residual* - one of those statistical terms that bring on the sweats. It refers to the residual difference left over after the line is fitted.

You can use the simple regression Shiny app[2] to explore the concept. We want the residuals to be as small as possible. We can square each residual (to get rid of minuses and make the algebra more convenient) and add them up. If this number is as small as possible, the line is fitting as best it can. Or in more formal language, we want to minimise the sum of squared residuals.

The regression apps and example figures in this chapter have been adapted

---

[1] These data are created on the fly by the Shiny apps that are linked and explained in this chapter. This enables you to explore the different concepts using the same variables. For example, if you tell the multivariable app that coffee and smoking should be confounded, it will change the underlying dataset to conform. You can then investigate the output of the regression model to see how that corresponds to the "truth" (that in this case, you control).

[2] https://argoshare.is.ed.ac.uk/simple_regression

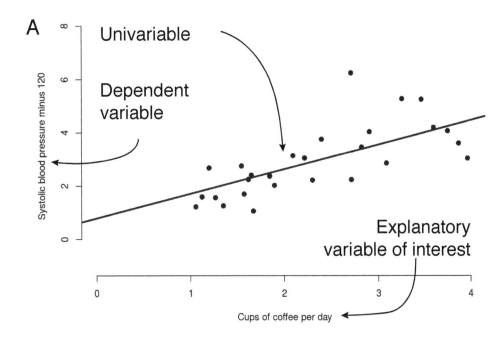

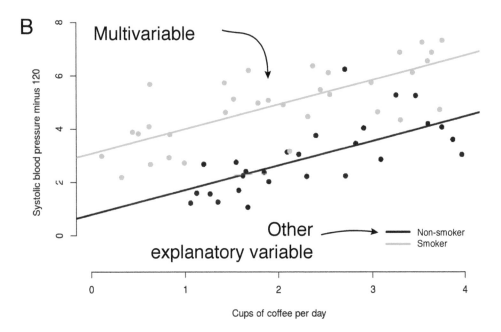

FIGURE 7.1: The anatomy of a regression plot. A - univariable linear regression, B - multivariable linear regression.

7.1.3   When the line fits well

Linear regression modelling has four main assumptions:

1. Linear relationship between predictors and outcome;
2. Independence of residuals;
3. Normal distribution of residuals;
4. Equal variance of residuals.

You can use the simple regression diagnostics shiny app[3] to get a handle on these.

Figure 7.3 shows diagnostic plots from the app, which we will run ourselves below Figure 7.13.

Linear relationship

A simple scatter plot should show a linear relationship between the explanatory and the dependent variable, as in Figure 7.3A. If the data describe a non-linear pattern (Figure 7.3B), then a straight line is not going to fit it well. In this situation, an alternative model should be considered, such as including a quadratic (squared, x^2) term.

Independence of residuals

The observations and therefore the residuals should be independent. This is more commonly a problem in time series data, where observations may be correlated across time with each other (autocorrelation).

Normal distribution of residuals

The observations should be normally distributed around the fitted line. This means that the residuals should show a normal distribution with a mean of zero (Figure 7.3A). If the observations are not equally distributed around the line, the histogram of residuals will be skewed and a normal Q-Q plot will show residuals diverging from the straight line (Figure 7.3B) (see Section 6.4.2).

Equal variance of residuals

The distance of the observations from the fitted line should be the same on the left side as on the right side. Look at the fan-shaped data on the simple

---

[3]`https://argoshare.is.ed.ac.uk/simple_regression_diagnostics`

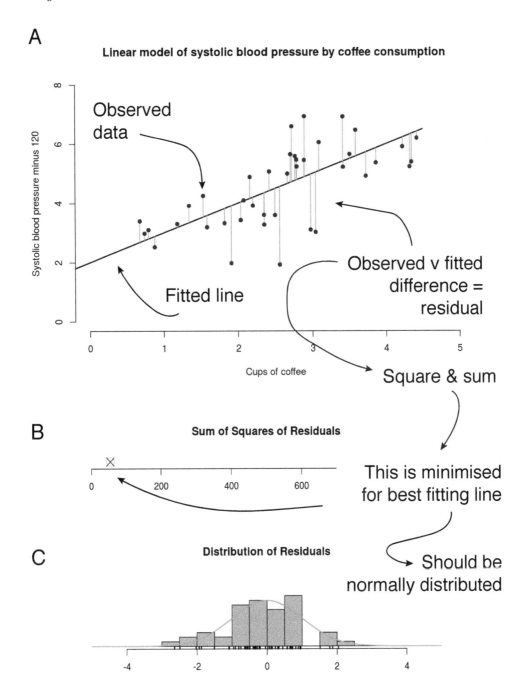

FIGURE 7.2: How a regression line is fitted. A - residuals are the green lines: the distance between each data point and the fitted line. B - the green circle indicates the minimum for these data; its absolute value is not meaningful or comparable with other datasets. Follow the "simple regression Shiny app" link to interact with the fitted line. A new sum of squares of residuals (the black cross) is calculated every time you move the line. C - Distribution of the residuals. App and plots adapted from https://github.com/mwaskom/ShinyApps with permission.

regression diagnostics Shiny app. This fan shape can be seen on the residuals vs fitted values plot.

Everything we talk about in this chapter is really about making sure that the line you draw through your data points is valid. It is about ensuring that the regression line is appropriate across the range of the explanatory variable and dependent variable. It is about understanding the underlying data, rather than relying on a fancy statistical test that gives you a p-value.

7.1.4   The fitted line and the linear equation

We promised to keep the equations to a minimum, but this one is so important it needs to be included. But it is easy to understand, so fear not.

Figure 7.4 links the fitted line, the linear equation, and the output from R. Some of this will likely be already familiar to you.

Figure 7.4A shows a scatter plot with fitted lines from a multivariable linear regression model. The plot is taken from the multivariable regression Shiny app[4]. Remember, these data are simulated and are not real. This app will really help you understand different regression models; more on this below. The app allows us to specify "the truth" with the sliders on the left-hand side. For instance, we can set the $intercept = 1$, meaning that when $x = 0$, the value of the dependent variable, $y = 1$.

Our model has a continuous explanatory variable of interest (average coffee consumption) and a further categorical variable (smoking). In the example the truth is set as $intercept = 1$, $\beta_1 = 1$ (true effect of coffee on blood pressure, slope of line), and $\beta_2 = 2$ (true effect of smoking on blood pressure). The points on the plot are simulated and include random noise.

What does $\beta_1 = 1$ mean? This is the slope of the line. So for each unit on the x-axis, there is a corresponding increase of one unit on the y-axis.

Figure 7.4B shows the default output in R for this linear regression model. Look carefully and make sure you are clear how the fitted lines, the linear equation, and the R output fit together. In this example, the random sample from our true population specified above shows $intercept = 0.67$, $\beta_1 = 1.00$ (coffee), and $\beta_2 = 2.48$ (smoking). A p-value is provided ($Pr(> |t|)$), which is the result of a null hypothesis significance test for the slope of the line being equal to zero.

---

[4]https://argoshare.is.ed.ac.uk/multi_regression/

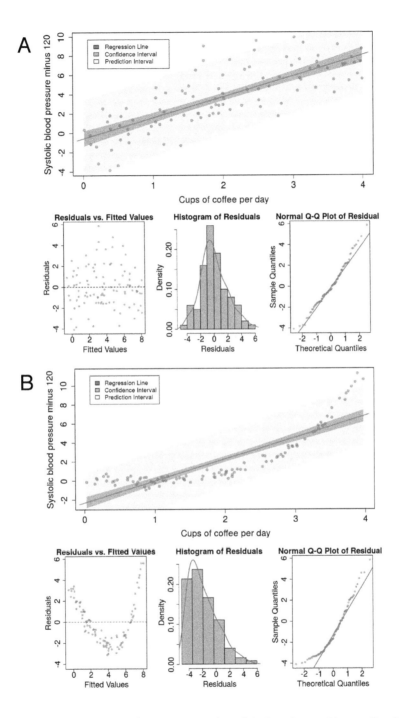

FIGURE 7.3: Regression diagnostics. A - this is what a linear fit should look like. B - this is not approriate; a non-linear model should be used instead. App and plots adapted from https://github.com/ShinyEd/intro-stats with permission.

A

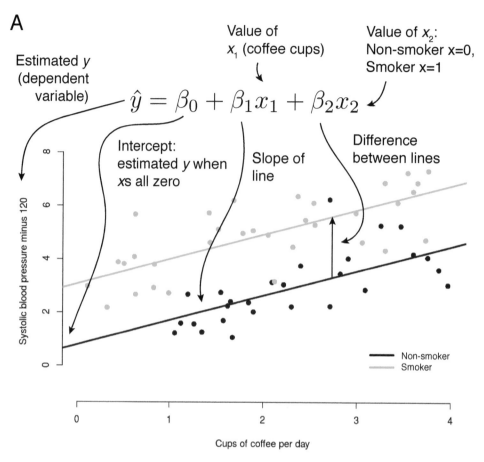

B   Linear regression (`lm`) output

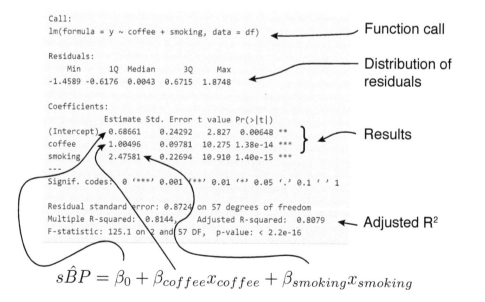

FIGURE 7.4: Linking the fitted line, regression equation and R output.

7.1.5 Effect modification

Effect modification occurs when the size of the effect of the explanatory variable of interest (exposure) on the outcome (dependent variable) differs depending on the level of a third variable. Said another way, this is a situation in which an explanatory variable differentially (positively or negatively) modifies the observed effect of another explanatory variable on the outcome.

Figure 7.5 shows three potential causal pathways using examples from the multivariable regression Shiny app[5].

In the first, smoking is not associated with the outcome (blood pressure) or our explanatory variable of interest (coffee consumption).

In the second, smoking is associated with elevated blood pressure, but not with coffee consumption. This is an example of effect modification.

In the third, smoking is associated with elevated blood pressure and with coffee consumption. This is an example of confounding.

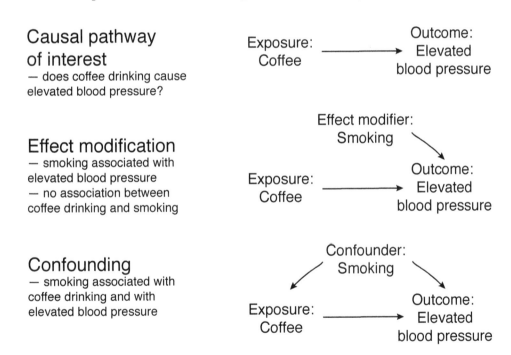

FIGURE 7.5: Causal pathways, effect modification and confounding.

Additive vs. multiplicative effect modification (interaction)

The name for these concepts differs depending on the field you work in. Effect

---

[5]https://argoshare.is.ed.ac.uk/multi_regression/

modification can be additive or multiplicative. We can refer to multiplicative effect modification as "a statistical interaction".

Figure 7.6 should make it clear exactly how these work. The data have been set up to include an interaction between the two explanatory variables. What does this mean?

- *intercept* $= 1$: the blood pressure $(\hat{y})$ for non-smokers who drink no coffee (all $x = 0$);
- $\beta_1 = 1$ (coffee): the additional blood pressure for each cup of coffee drunk by non-smokers (slope of the line when $x_2 = 0$);
- $\beta_2 = 1$ (smoking): the difference in blood pressure between non-smokers and smokers who drink no coffee ($x_1 = 0$);
- $\beta_3 = 1$ (coffee:smoking interaction): the blood pressure $(\hat{y})$ in addition to β_1 and β_2, for each cup of coffee drunk by smokers ($x_2 = 1$).

You may have to read that a couple of times in combination with looking at Figure 7.6.

With the additive model, the fitted lines for non-smoking vs smoking must always be parallel (the statistical term is 'constrained'). Look at the equation in Figure 7.6B and convince yourself that the lines can never be anything other than parallel.

A statistical interaction (or multiplicative effect modification) is a situation where the effect of an explanatory variable on the outcome is modified in non-additive manner. In other words using our example, the fitted lines are no longer constrained to be parallel.

If we had not checked for an interaction effect, we would have inadequately described the true relationship between these three variables.

What does this mean back in reality? Well it may be biologically plausible for the effect of smoking on blood pressure to increase multiplicatively due to a chemical interaction between cigarette smoke and caffeine, for example.

Note, we are just trying to find a model which best describes the underlying data. All models are approximations of reality.

7.1.6   R-squared and model fit

Figure 7.6 includes a further metric from the R output: Adjusted R-squared.

R-squared is another measure of how close the data are to the fitted line. It is also known as the *coefficient of determination* and represents the proportion of the dependent variable which is explained by the explanatory variable(s). So 0.0 indicates that none of the variability in the dependent is explained by

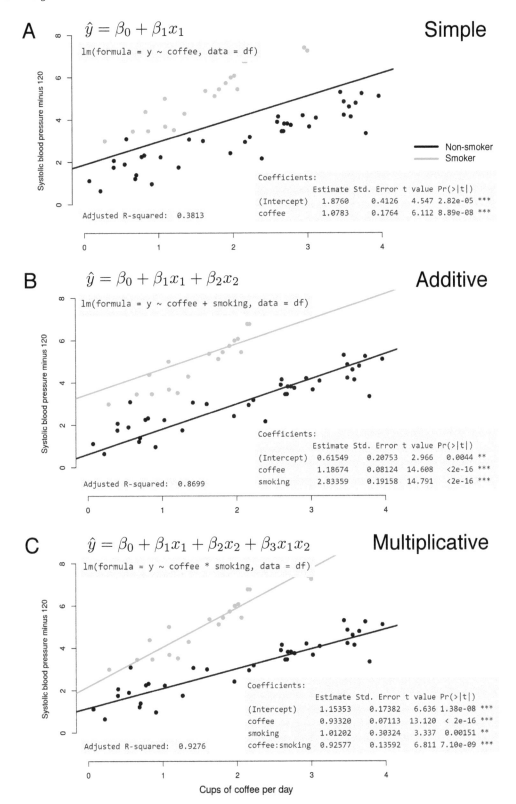

FIGURE 7.6: Multivariable linear regression with additive and multiplicative effect modification.

the explanatory (no relationship between data points and fitted line) and 1.0 indicates that the model explains all of the variability in the dependent (fitted line follows data points exactly).

R provides the R-squared and the Adjusted R-squared. The adjusted R-squared includes a penalty the more explanatory variables are included in the model. So if the model includes variables which do not contribute to the description of the dependent variable, the adjusted R-squared will be lower.

Looking again at Figure 7.6, in A, a simple model of coffee alone does not describe the data well (adjusted R-squared 0.38). Adding smoking to the model improves the fit as can be seen by the fitted lines (0.87). But a true interaction exists in the actual data. By including this interaction in the model, the fit is very good indeed (0.93).

7.1.7   Confounding

The last important concept to mention here is confounding. Confounding is a situation in which the association between an explanatory variable (exposure) and outcome (dependent variable) is distorted by the presence of another explanatory variable.

In our example, confounding exists if there is an association between smoking and blood pressure AND smoking and coffee consumption (Figure 7.5C). This exists if smokers drink more coffee than non-smokers.

Figure 7.7 shows this really clearly. The underlying data have now been altered so that those who drink more than two cups of coffee per day also smoke and those who drink fewer than two cups per day do not smoke. A true effect of smoking on blood pressure is simulated, but there is NO effect of coffee on blood pressure in this example.

If we only fit blood pressure by coffee consumption (Figure 7.7A), then we may mistakenly conclude a relationship between coffee consumption and blood pressure. But this does not exist, because the ground truth we have set is that no relationship exists between coffee and blood pressure. We are actually looking at the effect of smoking on blood pressure, which is confounding the effect of coffee on blood pressure.

If we include the confounder in the model by adding smoking, the true relationship becomes apparent. Two parallel flat lines indicating no effect of coffee on blood pressure, but a relationship between smoking and blood pressure. This procedure is referred to as controlling for or adjusting for confounders.

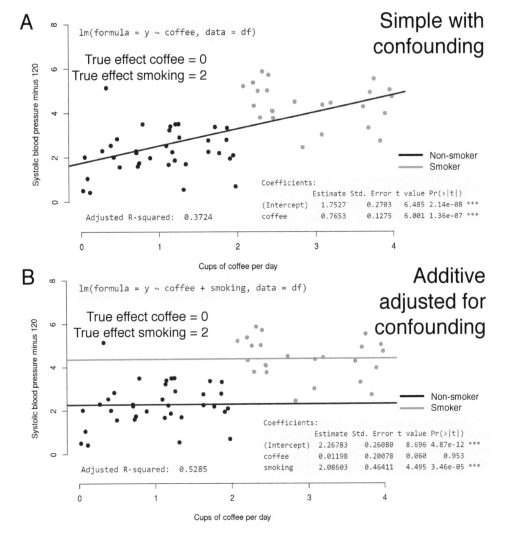

FIGURE 7.7: Multivariable linear regression with confounding of coffee drinking by smoking.

7.1.8 Summary

We have intentionally spent some time going through the principles and applications of linear regression because it is so important. A firm grasp of these concepts leads to an understanding of other regression procedures, such as logistic regression and Cox Proportional Hazards regression.

We will now perform all this ourselves in R using the gapminder dataset which you are familiar with from preceding chapters.

7.2   Fitting simple models

7.2.1   The Question (2)

We are interested in modelling the change in life expectancy for different countries over the past 60 years.

7.2.2   Get the data

```
library(tidyverse)
library(gapminder) # dataset
library(finalfit)
library(broom)

theme_set(theme_bw())
gapdata <- gapminder
```

7.2.3   Check the data

Always check a new dataset, as described in Section 6.3.

```
glimpse(gapdata) # each variable as line, variable type, first values
missing_glimpse(gapdata) # missing data for each variable
ff_glimpse(gapdata) # summary statistics for each variable
```

7.2.4   Plot the data

Let's plot the life expectancies in European countries over the past 60 years, focussing on the UK and Turkey. We can add in simple best fit lines using geom_smooth().

```
gapdata %>%
  filter(continent == "Europe") %>%    # Europe only
  ggplot(aes(x = year, y = lifeExp)) + # lifeExp~year
  geom_point() +                       # plot points
  facet_wrap(~ country) +              # facet by country
  scale_x_continuous(
    breaks = c(1960, 2000)) +          # adjust x-axis
  geom_smooth(method = "lm")           # add regression lines

## `geom_smooth()` using formula 'y ~ x'
```

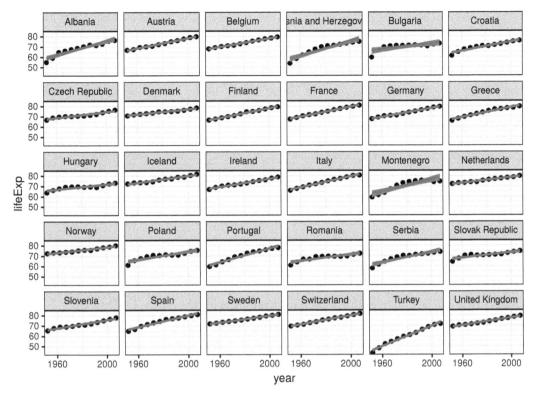

FIGURE 7.8: Scatter plots with linear regression lines: Life expectancy by year in European countries.

7.2.5 Simple linear regression

As you can see, `ggplot()` is very happy to run and plot linear regression models for us. While this is convenient for a quick look, we usually want to build, run, and explore these models ourselves. We can then investigate the intercepts and the slope coefficients (linear increase per year):

First let's plot two countries to compare, Turkey and United Kingdom:

```
gapdata %>%
  filter(country %in% c("Turkey", "United Kingdom")) %>%
  ggplot(aes(x = year, y = lifeExp, colour = country)) +
  geom_point()
```

The two non-parallel lines may make you think of what has been discussed above (Figure 7.6).

First, let's model the two countries separately.

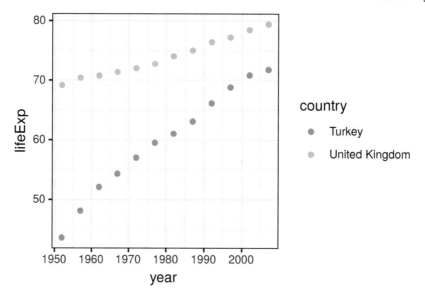

FIGURE 7.9: Scatter plot: Life expectancy by year: Turkey and United Kingdom

```
# United Kingdom
fit_uk <- gapdata %>%
  filter(country == "United Kingdom") %>%
  lm(lifeExp~year, data = .)

fit_uk %>%
  summary()


##
## Call:
## lm(formula = lifeExp ~ year, data = .)
##
## Residuals:
##      Min       1Q   Median       3Q      Max
## -0.69767 -0.31962  0.06642  0.36601  0.68165
##
## Coefficients:
##                Estimate Std. Error t value Pr(>|t|)
## (Intercept) -2.942e+02  1.464e+01  -20.10 2.05e-09 ***
## year         1.860e-01  7.394e-03   25.15 2.26e-10 ***
## ---
## Signif. codes:  0 '***' 0.001 '**' 0.01 '*' 0.05 '.' 0.1 ' ' 1
##
## Residual standard error: 0.4421 on 10 degrees of freedom
## Multiple R-squared:  0.9844, Adjusted R-squared:  0.9829
## F-statistic: 632.5 on 1 and 10 DF,  p-value: 2.262e-10


# Turkey
fit_turkey <- gapdata %>%
  filter(country == "Turkey") %>%
  lm(lifeExp~year, data = .)
```

```
fit_turkey %>%
  summary()
```

```
##
## Call:
## lm(formula = lifeExp ~ year, data = .)
##
## Residuals:
##     Min      1Q  Median      3Q     Max
## -2.4373 -0.3457  0.1653  0.9008  1.1033
##
## Coefficients:
##              Estimate Std. Error t value Pr(>|t|)
## (Intercept) -924.58989   37.97715  -24.35 3.12e-10 ***
## year           0.49724    0.01918   25.92 1.68e-10 ***
## ---
## Signif. codes:  0 '***' 0.001 '**' 0.01 '*' 0.05 '.' 0.1 ' ' 1
##
## Residual standard error: 1.147 on 10 degrees of freedom
## Multiple R-squared:  0.9853, Adjusted R-squared:  0.9839
## F-statistic: 671.8 on 1 and 10 DF,  p-value: 1.681e-10
```

Accessing the coefficients of linear regression

A simple linear regression model will return two coefficients - the intercept and the slope (the second returned value). Compare these coefficients to the `summary()` output above to see where these numbers came from.

```
fit_uk$coefficients
```

```
## (Intercept)        year
## -294.1965876   0.1859657
```

```
fit_turkey$coefficients
```

```
## (Intercept)        year
## -924.5898865   0.4972399
```

The slopes make sense - the results of the linear regression say that in the UK, life expectancy increases by 0.186 every year, whereas in Turkey the change is 0.497 per year. The reason the intercepts are negative, however, may be less obvious.

In this example, the intercept is telling us that life expectancy at year 0 in the United Kingdom (some 2000 years ago) was -294 years. While this is mathematically correct (based on the data we have), it obviously makes no sense in practice. It is important to think about the range over which you can extend your model predictions, and where they just become unrealistic.

To make the intercepts meaningful, we will add in a new column called
`year_from1952` and re-run `fit_uk` and `fit_turkey` using `year_from1952` instead of `year`.

```
gapdata <- gapdata %>%
  mutate(year_from1952 = year - 1952)

fit_uk <- gapdata %>%
  filter(country == "United Kingdom") %>%
  lm(lifeExp ~ year_from1952, data = .)

fit_turkey <- gapdata %>%
  filter(country == "Turkey") %>%
  lm(lifeExp ~ year_from1952, data = .)
```

```
fit_uk$coefficients
```

```
##   (Intercept) year_from1952
##    68.8085256     0.1859657
```

```
fit_turkey$coefficients
```

```
##   (Intercept) year_from1952
##    46.0223205     0.4972399
```

Now, the updated results tell us that in year 1952, the life expectancy in the
United Kingdom was 69 years. Note that the slopes do not change. There
was nothing wrong with the original model and the results were correct, the
intercept was just not meaningful.

Accessing all model information `tidy()` and `glance()`

In the fit_uk and fit_turkey examples above, we were using `fit_uk %>% summary()`
to get R to print out a summary of the model. This summary is not, however,
in a rectangular shape so we can't easily access the values or put them in a
table/use as information on plot labels.

We use the `tidy()` function from `library(broom)` to get the variable(s) and specific
values in a nice tibble:

```
fit_uk %>% tidy()
```

```
## # A tibble: 2 x 5
##   term          estimate std.error statistic  p.value
##   <chr>            <dbl>     <dbl>     <dbl>    <dbl>
## 1 (Intercept)      68.8     0.240     287.  6.58e-21
## 2 year_from1952    0.186   0.00739    25.1  2.26e-10
```

In the `tidy()` output, the column `estimate` includes both the intercepts and
slopes.

And we use the `glance()` function to get overall model statistics (mostly the r.squared).

```
fit_uk %>% glance()
```

```
## # A tibble: 1 x 12
##   r.squared adj.r.squared sigma statistic  p.value    df logLik   AIC   BIC
##       <dbl>         <dbl> <dbl>     <dbl>    <dbl> <dbl>  <dbl> <dbl> <dbl>
## 1     0.984         0.983 0.442      633. 2.26e-10     1  -6.14  18.3  19.7
## # ... with 3 more variables: deviance <dbl>, df.residual <int>, nobs <int>
```

7.2.6   Multivariable linear regression

Multivariable linear regression includes more than one explanatory variable. There are a few ways to include more variables, depending on whether they should share the intercept and how they interact:

Simple linear regression (exactly one predictor variable):

```
myfit = lm(lifeExp ~ year, data = gapdata)
```

Multivariable linear regression (additive):

```
myfit = lm(lifeExp ~ year + country, data = gapdata)
```

Multivariable linear regression (interaction):

```
myfit = lm(lifeExp ~ year * country, data = gapdata)
```

This equivalent to: `myfit = lm(lifeExp ~ year + country + year:country, data = gapdata)`

These examples of multivariable regression include two variables: `year` and `country`, but we could include more by adding them with `+`, it does not just have to be two.

We will now create three different linear regression models to further illustrate the difference between a simple model, additive model, and multiplicative model.

Model 1: year only

```
# UK and Turkey dataset
gapdata_UK_T <- gapdata %>%
  filter(country %in% c("Turkey", "United Kingdom"))

fit_both1 <- gapdata_UK_T %>%
  lm(lifeExp ~ year_from1952, data = .)
fit_both1
```

```
##
## Call:
## lm(formula = lifeExp ~ year_from1952, data = .)
```

```
##
## Coefficients:
##   (Intercept)   year_from1952
##       57.4154          0.3416
```

```
gapdata_UK_T %>%
  mutate(pred_lifeExp = predict(fit_both1)) %>%
  ggplot() +
  geom_point(aes(x = year, y = lifeExp, colour = country)) +
  geom_line(aes(x = year, y = pred_lifeExp))
```

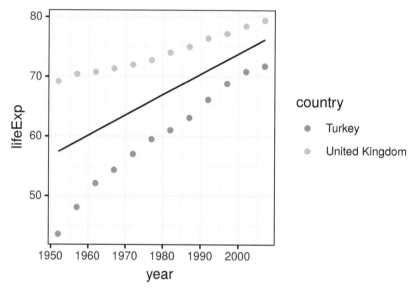

FIGURE 7.10: Scatter and line plot. Life expectancy in Turkey and the UK - univariable fit.

By fitting to year only (`lifeExp ~ year_from1952`), the model ignores country. This gives us a fitted line which is the average of life expectancy in the UK and Turkey. This may be desirable, depending on the question. But here we want to best describe the data.

How we made the plot and what does `predict()` do? Previously, we were using `geom_smooth(method = "lm")` to conveniently add linear regression lines on a scatter plot. When a scatter plot includes categorical value (e.g., the points are coloured by a variable), the regression lines `geom_smooth()` draws are multiplicative. That is great, and almost always exactly what we want. Here, however, to illustrate the difference between the different models, we will have to use the `predict()` model and `geom_line()` to have full control over the plotted regression lines.

```
gapdata_UK_T %>%
  mutate(pred_lifeExp = predict(fit_both1)) %>%
  select(country, year, lifeExp, pred_lifeExp) %>%
  group_by(country) %>%
  slice(1, 6, 12)
```

```
## # A tibble: 6 x 4
## # Groups:    country [2]
##    country         year lifeExp pred_lifeExp
##    <fct>          <int>   <dbl>        <dbl>
## 1 Turkey          1952    43.6         57.4
## 2 Turkey          1977    59.5         66.0
## 3 Turkey          2007    71.8         76.2
## 4 United Kingdom  1952    69.2         57.4
## 5 United Kingdom  1977    72.8         66.0
## 6 United Kingdom  2007    79.4         76.2
```

Note how the `slice()` function recognises group_by() and in this case shows us the 1st, 6th, and 12th observation within each group.

Model 2: year + country

```
fit_both2 <- gapdata_UK_T %>%
  lm(lifeExp ~ year_from1952 + country, data = .)
fit_both2
```

```
##
## Call:
## lm(formula = lifeExp ~ year_from1952 + country, data = .)
##
## Coefficients:
##          (Intercept)        year_from1952  countryUnited Kingdom
##              50.3023               0.3416                14.2262
```

```
gapdata_UK_T %>%
  mutate(pred_lifeExp = predict(fit_both2)) %>%
  ggplot() +
  geom_point(aes(x = year, y = lifeExp, colour = country)) +
  geom_line(aes(x = year, y = pred_lifeExp, colour = country))
```

This is better, by including country in the model, we now have fitted lines more closely representing the data. However, the lines are constrained to be parallel. This is the additive model that was discussed above. We need to include an interaction term to allow the effect of year on life expectancy to vary by country in a non-additive manner.

*Model 3: year * country*

```
fit_both3 <- gapdata_UK_T %>%
  lm(lifeExp ~ year_from1952 * country, data = .)
fit_both3
```

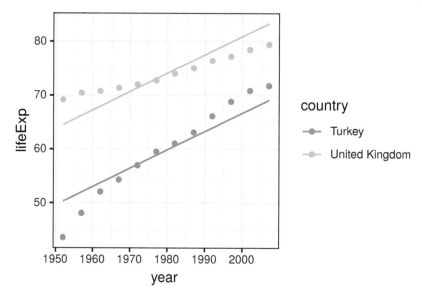

FIGURE 7.11: Scatter and line plot. Life expectancy in Turkey and the UK - multivariable additive fit.

```
##
## Call:
## lm(formula = lifeExp ~ year_from1952 * country, data = .)
##
## Coefficients:
##                       (Intercept)                        year_from1952
##                           46.0223                               0.4972
##            countryUnited Kingdom  year_from1952:countryUnited Kingdom
##                           22.7862                              -0.3113
```

```
gapdata_UK_T %>%
  mutate(pred_lifeExp = predict(fit_both3)) %>%
  ggplot() +
  geom_point(aes(x = year, y = lifeExp, colour = country)) +
  geom_line(aes(x = year, y = pred_lifeExp, colour = country))
```

This fits the data much better than the previous two models. You can check the R-squared using `summary(fit_both3)`.

Advanced tip: we can apply a function on multiple objects at once by putting them in a `list()` and using a `map_()` function from the **purrr** package. `library(purrr)` gets installed and loaded with `library(tidyverse)`, but it is outside the scope of this book. Do look it up once you get a little more comfortable with using R, and realise that you are starting to do similar things over and over again. For example, this code:

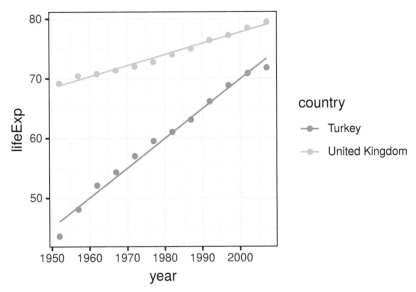

FIGURE 7.12: Scatter and line plot. Life expectancy in Turkey and the UK - multivariable multiplicative fit.

```
mod_stats1 <- glance(fit_both1)
mod_stats2 <- glance(fit_both2)
mod_stats3 <- glance(fit_both3)

bind_rows(mod_stats1, mod_stats2, mod_stats3)
```

returns the exact same thing as:

```
list(fit_both1, fit_both2, fit_both3) %>%
  map_df(glance)
```

```
## # A tibble: 3 x 12
##   r.squared adj.r.squared sigma statistic  p.value    df logLik   AIC   BIC
##       <dbl>         <dbl> <dbl>     <dbl>    <dbl> <dbl>  <dbl> <dbl> <dbl>
## 1     0.373         0.344  7.98      13.1 1.53e- 3     1  -82.9 172.  175.
## 2     0.916         0.908  2.99     114.  5.18e-12     2  -58.8 126.  130.
## 3     0.993         0.992 0.869     980.  7.30e-22     3  -28.5  67.0  72.9
## # ... with 3 more variables: deviance <dbl>, df.residual <int>, nobs <int>
```

What happens here is that `map_df()` applies a function on each object in the list it gets passed, and returns a df (data frame). In this case, the function is `glance()` (note that once inside `map_df()`, `glance` does not have its own brackets.

7.2.7 Check assumptions

The assumptions of linear regression can be checked with diagnostic plots, either by passing the fitted object (`lm()` output) to base R `plot()`, or by using the more convenient function below.

```
library(ggfortify)
autoplot(fit_both3)
```

```
## Warning: `arrange_()` is deprecated as of dplyr 0.7.0.
## Please use `arrange()` instead.
## See vignette('programming') for more help
## This warning is displayed once every 8 hours.
## Call `lifecycle::last_warnings()` to see where this warning was generated.
```

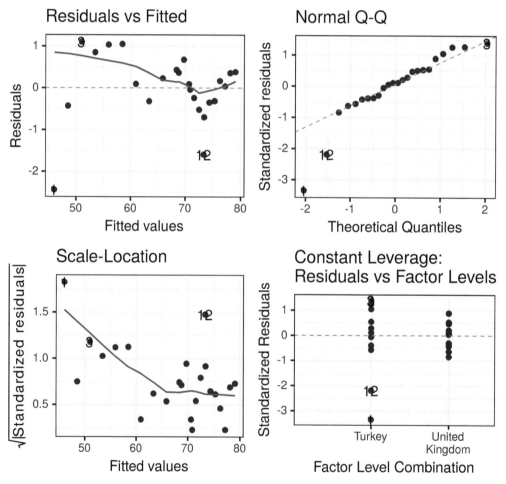

FIGURE 7.13: Diagnostic plots. Life expectancy in Turkey and the UK - multivariable multiplicative model.

7.3 Fitting more complex models

7.3.1 The Question (3)

Finally in this section, we are going to fit a more complex linear regression model. Here, we will discuss variable selection and introduce the Akaike Information Criterion (AIC).

We will introduce a new dataset: The Western Collaborative Group Study. This classic dataset includes observations of 3154 healthy young men aged 39-59 from the San Francisco area who were assessed for their personality type. It aimed to capture the occurrence of coronary heart disease over the following 8.5 years.

We will use it, however, to explore the relationship between systolic blood pressure (sbp) and personality type (personality_2L), accounting for potential confounders such as weight (weight). Now this is just for fun - don't write in!

The study was designed to look at cardiovascular events as the outcome, not blood pressure. But it is convenient to use blood pressure as a continuous outcome from this dataset, even if that was not the intention of the study.

The included personality types are A: aggressive and B: passive.

7.3.2 Model fitting principles

We suggest building statistical models on the basis of the following six pragmatic principles:

1. As few explanatory variables should be used as possible (parsimony);
2. Explanatory variables associated with the outcome variable in previous studies should be accounted for;
3. Demographic variables should be included in model exploration;
4. Population stratification should be incorporated if available;
5. Interactions should be checked and included if influential;
6. Final model selection should be performed using a "criterion-based approach"

- minimise the Akaike information criterion (AIC)
- maximise the adjusted R-squared value.

This is not the law, but it probably should be. These principles are sensible as we will discuss through the rest of this book. We strongly suggest you do not use automated methods of variable selection. These are often "forward selection" or "backward elimination" methods for including or excluding particular variables on the basis of a statistical property.

In certain settings, these approaches may be found to work. However, they create an artificial distance between you and the problem you are working on. They give you a false sense of certainty that the model you have created is in some sense valid. And quite frequently, they will just get it wrong.

Alternatively, you can follow the six principles above.

A variable may have previously been shown to strongly predict an outcome (think smoking and risk of cancer). This should give you good reason to consider it in your model. But perhaps you think that previous studies were incorrect, or that the variable is confounded by another. All this is fair, but it will be expected that this new knowledge is clearly demonstrated by you, so do not omit these variables before you start.

There are some variables that are so commonly associated with particular outcomes in healthcare that they should almost always be included at the start. Age, sex, social class, and co-morbidity for instance are commonly associated with survival. These need to be assessed before you start looking at your explanatory variable of interest.

Furthermore, patients are often clustered by a particular grouping variable, such as treating hospital. There will be commonalities between these patients that may not be fully explained by your observed variables. To estimate the coefficients of your variables of interest most accurately, clustering should be accounted for in the analysis.

As demonstrated above, the purpose of the model is to provide a best fit approximation of the underlying data. Effect modification and interactions commonly exist in health datasets, and should be incorporated if present.

Finally, we want to assess how well our models fit the data with 'model checking'. The effect of adding or removing one variable to the coefficients of the other variables in the model is very important, and will be discussed later. Measures of goodness-of-fit such as the AIC, can also be of great use when deciding which model choice is most valid.

7.3.3   AIC

The Akaike Information Criterion (AIC) is an alternative goodness-of-fit measure. In that sense, it is similar to the R-squared, but it has a different statistical basis. It is useful because it can be used to help guide the best fit in generalised linear models such as logistic regression (see Chapter 9). It is based on the likelihood but is also penalised for the number of variables present in the model. We aim to have as small an AIC as possible. The value of the number itself has no inherent meaning, but it is used to compare different models of the same data.

7.3.4 Get the data

```
wcgsdata <- finalfit::wcgs #press F1 here for details
```

7.3.5 Check the data

As always, when you receive a new dataset, carefully check that it does not contain errors.

TABLE 7.1: WCGS data, ff_glimpse: continuous.

label	var_type	n	missing_n	mean	sd	median
Subject ID	<int>	3154	0	10477.9	5877.4	11405.5
Age (years)	<int>	3154	0	46.3	5.5	45.0
Height (inches)	<int>	3154	0	69.8	2.5	70.0
Weight (pounds)	<int>	3154	0	170.0	21.1	170.0
Systolic BP (mmHg)	<int>	3154	0	128.6	15.1	126.0
Diastolic BP (mmHg)	<int>	3154	0	82.0	9.7	80.0
Cholesterol (mg/100 ml)	<int>	3142	12	226.4	43.4	223.0
Cigarettes/day	<int>	3154	0	11.6	14.5	0.0
Time to CHD event	<int>	3154	0	2683.9	666.5	2942.0

TABLE 7.2: WCGS data, ff_glimpse: categorical.

label	var_type	n	missing_n	levels_n	levels	levels_count
Personality type	<fct>	3154	0	4	"A1" "A2" "B3" "B4"	264, 1325, 1216, 349
Personality type	<fct>	3154	0	2	"B" "A"	1565, 1589
Smoking	<fct>	3154	0	2	"Non-smoker" "Smoker"	1652, 1502
Corneal arcus	<fct>	3152	2	2	"No" "Yes" "(Missing)"	2211, 941, 2
CHD event	<fct>	3154	0	2	"No" "Yes"	2897, 257
Type CHD	<fct>	3154	0	4	"No" "MI_SD" "Silent_MI" "Angina"	2897, 135, 71, 51

7.3.6 Plot the data

```
wcgsdata %>%
   ggplot(aes(y = sbp, x = weight,
              colour = personality_2L)) +    # Personality type
   geom_point(alpha = 0.2) +                 # Add transparency
   geom_smooth(method = "lm", se = FALSE)
```

```
## `geom_smooth()` using formula 'y ~ x'
```

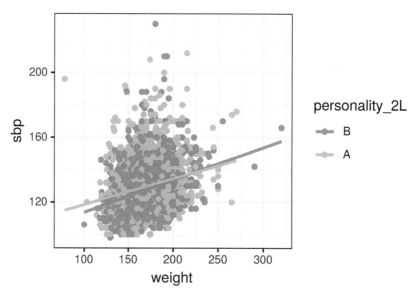

FIGURE 7.14: Scatter and line plot. Systolic blood pressure by weight and personality type.

From Figure 7.14, we can see that there is a weak relationship between weight and blood pressure.

In addition, there is really no meaningful effect of personality type on blood pressure. This is really important because, as you will see below, we are about to "find" some highly statistically significant effects in a model.

7.3.7 Linear regression with finalfit

finalfit is our own package and provides a convenient set of functions for fitting regression models with results presented in final tables.

There are a host of features with example code at the finalfit website[6].

Here we will use the all-in-one `finalfit()` function, which takes a dependent

---

[6]https://finalfit.org

variable and one or more explanatory variables. The appropriate regression for the dependent variable is performed, from a choice of linear, logistic, and Cox Proportional Hazards regression models. Summary statistics, together with a univariable and a multivariable regression analysis are produced in a final results table.

```
dependent <- "sbp"
explanatory <- "personality_2L"
fit_sbp1 <- wcgsdata %>%
  finalfit(dependent, explanatory, metrics = TRUE)
```

TABLE 7.3: Linear regression: Systolic blood pressure by personality type.

Dependent: Systolic BP (mmHg)	unit	value	Coefficient (univariable)	Coefficient (multivariable)
Personality type	B Mean (sd)	127.5 (14.4)	-	-
	A Mean (sd)	129.8 (15.7)	2.32 (1.26 to 3.37, p<0.001)	2.32 (1.26 to 3.37, p<0.001)

TABLE 7.4: Model metrics: Systolic blood pressure by personality type.

Number in dataframe = 3154, Number in model = 3154, Missing = 0, Log-likelihood = -13031.39, AIC = 26068.8, R-squared = 0.0059, Adjusted R-squared = 0.0056

Let's look first at our explanatory variable of interest, personality type. When a factor is entered into a regression model, the default is to compare each level of the factor with a "reference level". What you choose as the reference level can be easily changed (see Section 8.9. Alternative methods are available (sometimes called *contrasts*), but the default method is likely to be what you want almost all the time. Note this is sometimes referred to as creating a "dummy variable".

It can be seen that the mean blood pressure for type A is higher than for type B. As there is only one variable, the univariable and multivariable analyses are the same (the multivariable column can be removed if desired by including `select(-5) #5th column` in the piped function).

Although the difference is numerically quite small (2.3 mmHg), it is statistically significant partly because of the large number of patients in the study. The optional `metrics = TRUE` output gives us the number of rows (in this case, subjects) included in the model. This is important as frequently people forget that in standard regression models, missing data from any variable results in the entire row being excluded from the analysis (see Chapter 11).

Note the AIC and Adjusted R-squared results. The adjusted R-squared is very low - the model only explains only 0.6% of the variation in systolic blood pressure. This is to be expected, given our scatter plot above.

Let's now include subject weight, which we have hypothesised may influence blood pressure.

```
dependent <- "sbp"
explanatory <- c("weight", "personality_2L")
fit_sbp2 <- wcgsdata %>%
  finalfit(dependent, explanatory, metrics = TRUE)
```

TABLE 7.5: Multivariable linear regression: Systolic blood pressure by personality type and weight.

Dependent: Systolic BP (mmHg)	unit	value		Coefficient (univariable)	Coefficient (multivariable)
Weight (pounds)	[78.0,320.0]	Mean (sd)	128.6 (15.1)	0.18 (0.16 to 0.21, p<0.001)	0.18 (0.16 to 0.20, p<0.001)
Personality type	B	Mean (sd)	127.5 (14.4)	-	-
	A	Mean (sd)	129.8 (15.7)	2.32 (1.26 to 3.37, p<0.001)	1.99 (0.97 to 3.01, p<0.001)

TABLE 7.6: Multivariable linear regression metrics: Systolic blood pressure by personality type and weight.

Number in dataframe = 3154, Number in model = 3154, Missing = 0, Log-likelihood = -12928.82, AIC = 25865.6, R-squared = 0.068, Adjusted R-squared = 0.068

The output shows us the range for weight (78 to 320 pounds) and the mean (standard deviation) systolic blood pressure for the whole cohort.

The coefficient with 95% confidence interval is provided by default. This is interpreted as: for each pound increase in weight, there is on average a corresponding increase of 0.18 mmHg in systolic blood pressure.

Note the difference in the interpretation of continuous and categorical variables in the regression model output (Table 7.5).

The adjusted R-squared is now higher - the personality and weight together explain 6.8% of the variation in blood pressure.

The AIC is also slightly lower meaning this new model better fits the data.

There is little change in the size of the coefficients for each variable in the multivariable analysis, meaning that they are reasonably independent. As an exercise, check the distribution of weight by personality type using a boxplot.

Let's now add in other variables that may influence systolic blood pressure.

```
dependent <- "sbp"
explanatory <- c("personality_2L", "weight", "age",
                 "height", "chol", "smoking")
fit_sbp3 <- wcgsdata %>%
  finalfit(dependent, explanatory, metrics = TRUE)
```

TABLE 7.7: Multivariable linear regression: Systolic blood pressure by available explanatory variables.

Dependent: Systolic BP (mmHg)		unit	value	Coefficient (univariable)	Coefficient (multivariable)
Personality type	B	Mean (sd)	127.5 (14.4)	-	-
	A	Mean (sd)	129.8 (15.7)	2.32 (1.26 to 3.37, p<0.001)	1.44 (0.44 to 2.43, p=0.005)
Weight (pounds)	[78.0,320.0]	Mean (sd)	128.6 (15.1)	0.18 (0.16 to 0.21, p<0.001)	0.24 (0.21 to 0.27, p<0.001)
Age (years)	[39.0,59.0]	Mean (sd)	128.6 (15.1)	0.45 (0.36 to 0.55, p<0.001)	0.43 (0.33 to 0.52, p<0.001)
Height (inches)	[60.0,78.0]	Mean (sd)	128.6 (15.1)	0.11 (-0.10 to 0.32, p=0.302)	-0.84 (-1.08 to -0.61, p<0.001)
Cholesterol (mg/100 ml)	[103.0,645.0]	Mean (sd)	128.6 (15.1)	0.04 (0.03 to 0.05, p<0.001)	0.03 (0.02 to 0.04, p<0.001)
Smoking	Non-smoker	Mean (sd)	128.6 (15.6)	-	-
	Smoker	Mean (sd)	128.7 (14.6)	0.08 (-0.98 to 1.14, p=0.883)	0.95 (-0.05 to 1.96, p=0.063)

TABLE 7.8: Model metrics: Systolic blood pressure by available explanatory variables.

Number in dataframe = 3154, Number in model = 3142, Missing = 12, Log-likelihood = -12772.04, AIC = 25560.1, R-squared = 0.12, Adjusted R-squared = 0.12

Age, height, serum cholesterol, and smoking status have been added. Some of the variation explained by personality type has been taken up by these new variables - personality is now associated with an average change of blood pressure of 1.4 mmHg.

The adjusted R-squared now tells us that 12% of the variation in blood pressure is explained by the model, which is an improvement.

Look out for variables that show large changes in effect size or a change in the direction of effect when going from a univariable to multivariable model. This means that the other variables in the model are having a large effect on this variable and the cause of this should be explored. For instance, in this example the effect of height changes size and direction. This is because of the close association between weight and height. For instance, it may be more sensible to work with body mass index ($weight/height^2$) rather than the two separate variables.

In general, variables that are highly correlated with each other should be treated carefully in regression analysis. This is called collinearity and can lead to unstable estimates of coefficients. For more on this, see Section 9.4.2.

Let's create a new variable called bmi, note the conversion from pounds and inches to kg and m:

```
wcgsdata <- wcgsdata %>%
  mutate(
    bmi = ((weight*0.4536) / (height*0.0254)^2) %>%
      ff_label("BMI")
  )
```

Weight and height can now be replaced in the model with BMI.

```
explanatory <- c("personality_2L", "bmi", "age",
                 "chol", "smoking")

fit_sbp4 <- wcgsdata %>%
  finalfit(dependent, explanatory, metrics = TRUE)
```

TABLE 7.9: Multivariable linear regression: Systolic blood pressure using BMI.

Dependent: Systolic BP (mmHg)	unit	value		Coefficient (univariable)	Coefficient (multivariable)
Personality type	B	Mean (sd)	127.5 (14.4)	-	-
	A	Mean (sd)	129.8 (15.7)	2.32 (1.26 to 3.37, p<0.001)	1.51 (0.51 to 2.50, p=0.003)
BMI	[11.2,39.0]	Mean (sd)	128.6 (15.1)	1.69 (1.50 to 1.89, p<0.001)	1.65 (1.46 to 1.85, p<0.001)
Age (years)	[39.0,59.0]	Mean (sd)	128.6 (15.1)	0.45 (0.36 to 0.55, p<0.001)	0.41 (0.32 to 0.50, p<0.001)
Cholesterol (mg/100 ml)	[103.0,645.0]	Mean (sd)	128.6 (15.1)	0.04 (0.03 to 0.05, p<0.001)	0.03 (0.02 to 0.04, p<0.001)
Smoking	Non-smoker	Mean (sd)	128.6 (15.6)	-	-
	Smoker	Mean (sd)	128.7 (14.6)	0.08 (-0.98 to 1.14, p=0.883)	0.98 (-0.03 to 1.98, p=0.057)

TABLE 7.10: Model metrics: Systolic blood pressure using BMI.

Number in dataframe = 3154, Number in model = 3142, Missing = 12, Log-likelihood = -12775.03, AIC = 25564.1, R-squared = 0.12, Adjusted R-squared = 0.12

On the principle of parsimony, we may want to remove variables which are not contributing much to the model. For instance, let's compare models with and without the inclusion of smoking. This can be easily done using the `finalfit` `explanatory_multi` option.

```
dependent <- "sbp"
explanatory        <- c("personality_2L", "bmi", "age",
                        "chol", "smoking")
explanatory_multi <- c("bmi", "personality_2L", "age",
                       "chol")
fit_sbp5 <- wcgsdata %>%
  finalfit(dependent, explanatory,
           explanatory_multi,
           keep_models = TRUE, metrics = TRUE)
```

This results in little change in the other coefficients and very little change in the AIC. We will consider the reduced model the final model.

We can also visualise models using plotting. This is useful for communicating a model in a restricted space, e.g., in a presentation.

TABLE 7.11: Multivariable linear regression: Systolic blood pressure by available explanatory variables and reduced model.

Dependent: Systolic BP (mmHg)		unit	value	Coefficient (univariable)	Coefficient (multivariable)	Coefficient (multivariable reduced)
Personality type	B	Mean (sd)	127.5 (14.4)	-	-	-
	A	Mean (sd)	129.8 (15.7)	2.32 (1.26 to 3.37, p<0.001)	1.51 (0.51 to 2.50, p=0.003)	1.56 (0.57 to 2.56, p=0.002)
BMI	[11.2,39.0]	Mean (sd)	128.6 (15.1)	1.69 (1.50 to 1.89, p<0.001)	1.65 (1.46 to 1.85, p<0.001)	1.62 (1.43 to 1.82, p<0.001)
Age (years)	[39.0,59.0]	Mean (sd)	128.6 (15.1)	0.45 (0.36 to 0.55, p<0.001)	0.41 (0.32 to 0.50, p<0.001)	0.41 (0.32 to 0.50, p<0.001)
Cholesterol (mg/100 ml)	[103.0,645.0]	Mean (sd)	128.6 (15.1)	0.04 (0.03 to 0.05, p<0.001)	0.03 (0.02 to 0.04, p<0.001)	0.03 (0.02 to 0.04, p<0.001)
Smoking	Non-smoker	Mean (sd)	128.6 (15.6)	-	-	-
	Smoker	Mean (sd)	128.7 (14.6)	0.08 (-0.98 to 1.14, p=0.883)	0.98 (-0.03 to 1.98, p=0.057)	-

TABLE 7.12: Model metrics: Systolic blood pressure by available explanatory variables (top) with reduced model (bottom).

Number in dataframe = 3154, Number in model = 3142, Missing = 12, Log-likelihood = -12775.03, AIC = 25564.1, R-squared = 0.12, Adjusted R-squared = 0.12
Number in dataframe = 3154, Number in model = 3142, Missing = 12, Log-likelihood = -12776.83, AIC = 25565.7, R-squared = 0.12, Adjusted R-squared = 0.12

```
dependent <- "sbp"
explanatory          <- c("personality_2L", "bmi", "age",
                          "chol", "smoking")
explanatory_multi <- c("bmi", "personality_2L", "age",
                          "chol")
fit_sbp5 <- wcgsdata %>%
  ff_plot(dependent, explanatory_multi)
```

We can check the assumptions as above.

```
dependent <- "sbp"
explanatory_multi <- c("bmi", "personality_2L", "age",
                          "chol")
wcgsdata %>%
  lmmulti(dependent, explanatory_multi) %>%
  autoplot()
```

An important message in the results relates to the highly significant *p*-values in the table above. Should we conclude that in a multivariable regression model controlling for BMI, age, and serum cholesterol, blood pressure was significantly elevated in those with a Type A personality (1.56 (0.57 to 2.56, p=0.002) compared with Type B? The *p*-value looks impressive, but the actual difference in blood pressure is only 1.6 mmHg. Even at a population level, that may not be clinically significant, fitting with our first thoughts when we saw the scatter plot.

This serves to emphasise our most important point. Our focus should be on understanding the underlying data itself, rather than relying on complex mul-

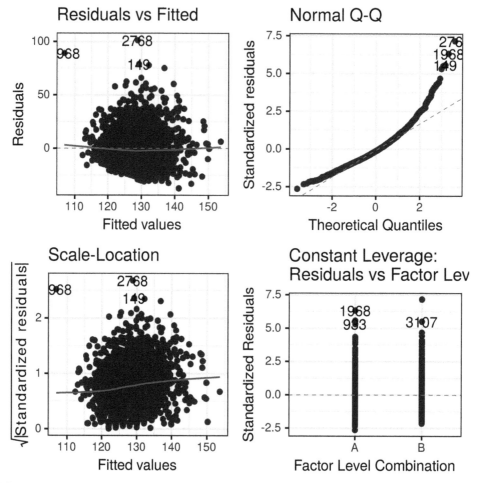

FIGURE 7.15: Diagnostic plots: Linear regression model of systolic blood pressure.

tidimensional modelling procedures. By making liberal use of upfront plotting, together with further visualisation as you understand the data, you will likely be able to draw most of the important conclusions that the data has to offer. Use modelling to quantify and confirm this, rather than as the primary method of data exploration.

7.3.8 Summary

Time spent truly understanding linear regression is well spent. Not because you will spend a lot of time making linear regression models in health data science (we rarely do), but because it the essential foundation for understanding more advanced statistical models.

It can even be argued that all common statistical tests are linear models[7]. This great post demonstrates beautifully how the statistical tests we are most familiar with (such as t-test, Mann-Whitney U test, ANOVA, chi-squared test) can simply be considered as special cases of linear models, or close approximations.

Regression is fitting lines, preferably straight, through data points. Make $\hat{y} = \beta_0 + \beta_1 x_1$ a close friend.

An excellent book for further reading on regression is Harrell (2015).

7.4 Exercises

7.4.1 Exercise

Using the multivariable regression Shiny app[8], hack some p-values to prove to yourself the principle of multiple testing.

From the default position, select "additive model" then set "Error standard deviation" to 2. Leave all true effects at 0. How many clicks of "New Sample" did you need before you got a statistically significant result?

7.4.2 Exercise

Plot the GDP per capita by year for countries in Europe. Add a best fit straight line to the plot. In which countries is the relationship not linear? Advanced: make the line curved by adding a quadratic/squared term, e.g., $y \; x^2 + x$. Hint: check geom_smooth() help page under formula.

7.4.3 Exercise

Compare the relationship between GDP per capita and year for two countries of your choice. If you can't choose, make it Albania and Austria.

Fit and plot a regression model that simply averages the values across the two countries.

Fit and plot a best fit regression model.

Use your model to determine the difference in GDP per capita for your countries in 1980.

---

[7] https://lindeloev.github.io/tests-as-linear
[8] https://argoshare.is.ed.ac.uk/multi_regression/

7.4.4 Exercise

Use the Western Collaborative Group Study data to determine if there is a relationship between age and cholesterol level.

Remember to plot the data first.

Make a simple regression model. Add other variables to adjust for potential confounding.

7.5 Solutions

Solution to Exercise 7.4.2:

```
gapdata %>%
  filter(continent == "Europe") %>%
  ggplot(aes(x = year, y = gdpPercap)) +
  geom_point() +
  geom_smooth(method = "lm") +
  facet_wrap(country ~ .)
```

```
## `geom_smooth()` using formula 'y ~ x'
```

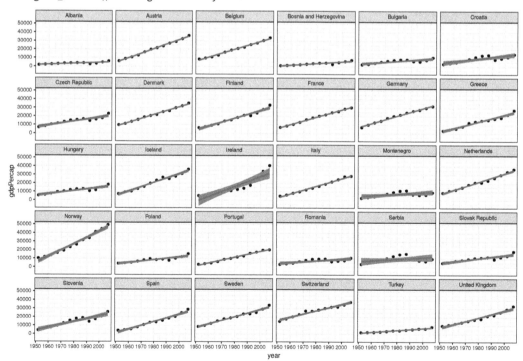

```
# Countries not linear: Ireland, Montenegro, Serbia.

# Add quadratic term
gapdata %>%
  filter(continent == "Europe") %>%
  ggplot(aes(x = year, y = gdpPercap)) +
  geom_point() +
  geom_smooth(method = "lm", formula = "y ~ poly(x, 2)") +
  facet_wrap(country ~ .)
```

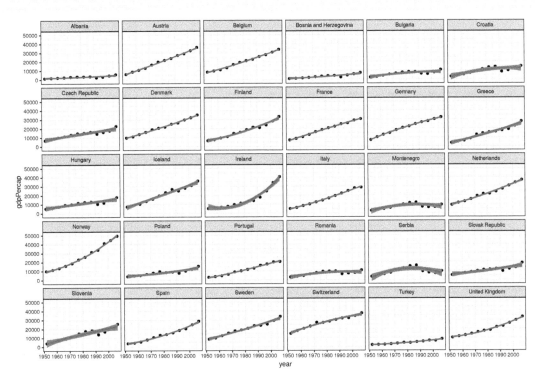

Solution to Exercise 7.4.3:

```
# Plot first
gapdata %>%
  filter(country %in% c("Albania", "Austria")) %>%
  ggplot() +
  geom_point(aes(x = year, y = gdpPercap, colour= country))
```

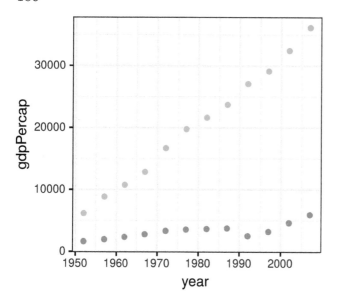

```
# Fit average line between two countries.
fit_both1 = gapdata %>%
    filter(country %in% c("Albania", "Austria")) %>%
    lm(gdpPercap ~ year, data = .)

gapdata %>%
    filter(country %in% c("Albania", "Austria")) %>%
    ggplot() +
    geom_point(aes(x = year, y = gdpPercap, colour = country)) +
    geom_line(aes(x = year, y = predict(fit_both1)))
```

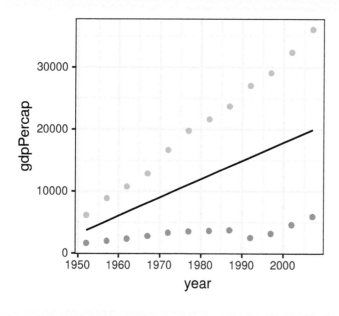

```
# Fit average line between two countries.
fit_both3 = gapdata %>%
    filter(country %in% c("Albania", "Austria")) %>%
```

```
  lm(gdpPercap ~ year * country, data = .)

gapdata %>%
  filter(country %in% c("Albania", "Austria")) %>%
  ggplot() +
  geom_point(aes(x = year, y = gdpPercap, colour = country)) +
  geom_line(aes(x = year, y = predict(fit_both3), group = country))
```

```
# You can use the regression equation by hand to work out the difference
summary(fit_both3)

# Or pass newdata to predict to estimate the two points of interest
gdp_1980 <- predict(fit_both3, newdata = data.frame(
  country = c("Albania", "Austria"),
  year = c(1980, 1980))
)
gdp_1980
gdp_1980[2] - gdp_1980[1]
```

Solution to Exercise 7.4.4:

```
# Plot data first
wcgsdata %>%
  ggplot(aes(x = age, y = chol))+
  geom_point() +
  geom_smooth(method = "lm", formula = "y~x")
```

```
## Warning: Removed 12 rows containing non-finite values (stat_smooth).

## Warning: Removed 12 rows containing missing values (geom_point).
```

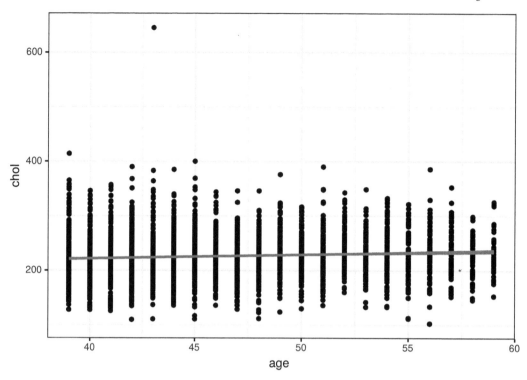

```
# Weak positive relationship

# Simple linear regression
dependent <- "chol"
explanatory <- "age"
wcgsdata %>%
  finalfit(dependent, explanatory, metrics = TRUE)
```

Note: dependent includes missing data. These are dropped.

```
# For each year of age, cholesterol increases by 0.7 mg/100 ml.
# This gradient differs from zero.

# Is this effect independent of other available variables?

# Make BMI as above
dependent <- "chol"
explanatory <- c( "age", "bmi", "sbp", "smoking", "personality_2L")
wcgsdata %>%
  mutate(
    bmi = ((weight*0.4536) / (height*0.0254)^2) %>%
      ff_label("BMI")
  ) %>%
  finalfit(dependent, explanatory, metrics = TRUE)
```

Note: dependent includes missing data. These are dropped.

```
# Effect size is reduced, but still present.
# Model poorly describes data, R2=0.033.
```

8

Working with categorical outcome variables

Suddenly Christopher Robin began to tell Pooh about some of the things:
People called Kings and Queens and something called Factors ... and Pooh
said "Oh!" and thought how wonderful it would be to have a Real Brain
which could tell you things.
A.A. Milne, *The House at Pooh Corner* (1928)

8.1 Factors

We said earlier that continuous data can be measured and categorical data
can be counted, which is useful to remember. Categorical data can be a:

- Factor
    - a fixed set of names/strings or numbers
    - these may have an inherent order (1st, 2nd 3rd) - ordinal factor
    - or may not (female, male)
- Character
    - sequences of letters, numbers, or symbols
- Logical
    - containing only TRUE or FALSE

Health data is awash with factors. Whether it is outcomes like death, recurrence, or readmission. Or predictors like cancer stage, deprivation quintile, or smoking status. It is essential therefore to be comfortable manipulating factors and dealing with outcomes which are categorical.

8.2   The Question

We will use the classic "Survival from Malignant Melanoma" dataset which is included in the **boot** package. The data consist of measurements made on patients with malignant melanoma, a type of skin cancer. Each patient had their tumour removed by surgery at the Department of Plastic Surgery, University Hospital of Odense, Denmark, between 1962 and 1977.

For the purposes of this discussion, we are interested in the association between tumour ulceration and death from melanoma.

8.3   Get the data

The Help page (F1 on `boot::melanoma`) gives us its data dictionary including the definition of each variable and the coding used.

```
meldata <- boot::melanoma
```

8.4   Check the data

As always, check any new dataset carefully before you start analysis.

```
library(tidyverse)
library(finalfit)
theme_set(theme_bw())
meldata %>% glimpse()
```

```
## Rows: 205
## Columns: 7
## $ time      <dbl> 10, 30, 35, 99, 185, 204, 210, 232, 232, 279, 295, 355, 3...
## $ status    <dbl> 3, 3, 2, 3, 1, 1, 1, 3, 1, 1, 1, 3, 1, 1, 1, 3, 1, 1, 1, ...
## $ sex       <dbl> 1, 1, 1, 0, 1, 1, 1, 0, 1, 0, 0, 0, 0, 1, 0, 1, 1, 1, 1, ...
## $ age       <dbl> 76, 56, 41, 71, 52, 28, 77, 60, 49, 68, 53, 64, 68, 63, 1...
## $ year      <dbl> 1972, 1968, 1977, 1968, 1965, 1971, 1972, 1974, 1968, 197...
## $ thickness <dbl> 6.76, 0.65, 1.34, 2.90, 12.08, 4.84, 5.16, 3.22, 12.88, 7...
## $ ulcer     <dbl> 1, 0, 0, 0, 1, 1, 1, 1, 1, 1, 1, 1, 1, 1, 1, 1, 1, 1, 1, ...
```

```
meldata %>% ff_glimpse()
```

```
## $Continuous
##                 label var_type   n missing_n missing_percent   mean     sd    min
## time             time    <dbl> 205         0             0.0 2152.8 1122.1   10.0
## status         status    <dbl> 205         0             0.0    1.8    0.6    1.0
## sex               sex    <dbl> 205         0             0.0    0.4    0.5    0.0
## age               age    <dbl> 205         0             0.0   52.5   16.7    4.0
## year             year    <dbl> 205         0             0.0 1969.9    2.6 1962.0
## thickness   thickness    <dbl> 205         0             0.0    2.9    3.0    0.1
## ulcer           ulcer    <dbl> 205         0             0.0    0.4    0.5    0.0
##             quartile_25 median quartile_75    max
## time             1525.0 2005.0      3042.0 5565.0
## status              1.0    2.0         2.0    3.0
## sex                 0.0    0.0         1.0    1.0
## age                42.0   54.0        65.0   95.0
## year             1968.0 1970.0      1972.0 1977.0
## thickness           1.0    1.9         3.6   17.4
## ulcer               0.0    0.0         1.0    1.0
##
## $Categorical
## data frame with 0 columns and 205 rows
```

As can be seen, all of the variables are currently coded as continuous/numeric. The `<dbl>` stands for 'double', meaning numeric which comes from 'double-precision floating point', an awkward computer science term.

8.5   Recode the data

It is really important that variables are correctly coded for all plotting and analysis functions. Using the data dictionary, we will convert the categorical variables to factors.

In the section below, we convert the continuous variables to `factors` (e.g., `sex %>% factor() %>%`), then use the **forcats** package to recode the factor levels. Modern databases (such as REDCap) can give you an R script to recode your specific dataset. This means you don't always have to recode your factors from numbers to names manually. But you will always be recoding variables during the exploration and analysis stages too, so it is important to follow what is happening here.

```
meldata <- meldata %>%
  mutate(sex.factor =          # Make new variable
           sex %>%             # from existing variable
           factor() %>%        # convert to factor
           fct_recode(         # forcats function
```

```
        "Female" = "0",       # new on left, old on right
        "Male"   = "1") %>%
    ff_label("Sex"),          # Optional label for finalfit

    # same thing but more condensed code:
    ulcer.factor = factor(ulcer) %>%
      fct_recode("Present" = "1",
                 "Absent"  = "0") %>%
      ff_label("Ulcerated tumour"),

    status.factor = factor(status) %>%
      fct_recode("Died melanoma"       = "1",
                 "Alive"               = "2",
                 "Died - other causes" = "3") %>%
      ff_label("Status"))
```

We have formatted the recode of the sex variables to be on multiple lines - to
make it easier for you to see the exact steps included. We have condensed for
the other recodes (e.g., ulcer.factor = factor(ulcer) %>%), but it does the exact
same thing as the first one.

8.6   Should I convert a continuous variable to a categorical variable?

This is a common question and something which is frequently done. Take for
instance the variable age. Is it better to leave it as a continuous variable, or
to chop it into categories, e.g., 30 to 39 etc.?

The clear disadvantage in doing this is that information is being thrown away.
Which feels like a bad thing to be doing. This is particularly important if the
categories being created are large.

For instance, if age was dichotomised to "young" and "old" at say 42 years
(the current median age in Europe), then it is likely that relevant information
to a number of analyses has been discarded.

Secondly, it is unforgivable practice to repeatedly try different cuts of a continuous variable to obtain a statistically significant result. This is most commonly
done in tests of diagnostic accuracy, where a threshold for considering a continuous test result positive is chosen *post hoc* to maximise sensitivity/specificity,
but not then validated in an independent cohort.

But there are also advantages to converting a continuous variable to categorical. Say the relationship between age and an outcome is not linear, but rather
u-shaped, then fitting a regression line is more difficult. If age is cut into 10-

year bands and entered into a regression as a factor, then this non-linearity is already accounted for.

Secondly, when communicating the results of an analysis to a lay audience, it may be easier to use a categorical representation. For instance, an odds of death 1.8 times greater in 70-year-olds compared with 40-year-olds may be easier to grasp than a 1.02 times increase per year.

So what is the answer? Do not do it unless you have to. Plot and understand the continuous variable first. If you do it, try not to throw away too much information. Repeat your analyses both with the continuous data and categorical data to ensure there is no difference in the conclusion (often called a sensitivity analysis).

```
# Summary of age
meldata$age %>%
  summary()
```

```
##    Min. 1st Qu.  Median    Mean 3rd Qu.    Max.
##    4.00   42.00   54.00   52.46   65.00   95.00
```

```
meldata %>%
  ggplot(aes(x = age)) +
  geom_histogram()
```

```
## `stat_bin()` using `bins = 30`. Pick better value with `binwidth`.
```

There are different ways in which a continuous variable can be converted to a factor. You may wish to create a number of intervals of equal length. The cut() function can be used for this.

Figure 8.1 illustrates different options for this. We suggest not using the label option of the cut() function to avoid errors, should the underlying data change or when the code is copied and reused. A better practice is to recode the levels using fct_recode as above.

The intervals in the output are standard mathematical notation. A square bracket indicates the value is included in the interval and a round bracket that the value is excluded.

Note the requirement for include.lowest = TRUE when you specify breaks yourself and the lowest cut-point is also the lowest data value. This should be clear in Figure 8.1.

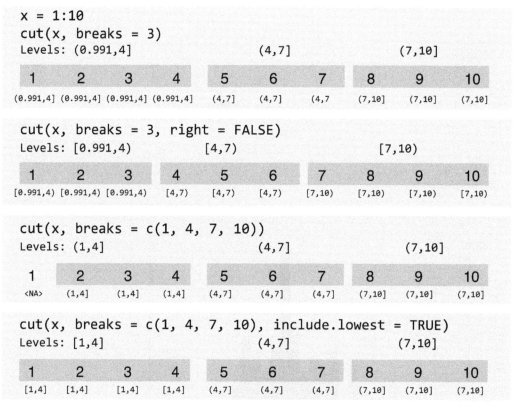

FIGURE 8.1: cut a continuous variable into a categorical variable.

8.6.1 Equal intervals vs quantiles

Be clear in your head whether you wish to cut the data so the intervals are of equal length. Or whether you wish to cut the data so there are equal proportions of cases (patients) in each level.

Equal intervals:

```
meldata <- meldata %>%
  mutate(
    age.factor =
      age %>%
      cut(4)
  )
meldata$age.factor %>%
  summary()
```

```
## (3.91,26.8] (26.8,49.5] (49.5,72.2] (72.2,95.1]
##          16          68         102          19
```

Quantiles:

```
meldata <- meldata %>%
  mutate(
    age.factor =
      age %>%
      Hmisc::cut2(g=4) # Note, cut2 comes from the Hmisc package
  )
meldata$age.factor %>%
  summary()
```

```
## [ 4,43) [43,55) [55,66) [66,95]
##      55      49      53      48
```

Using the cut function, a continuous variable can be converted to a categorical one:

```
meldata <- meldata %>%
  mutate(
    age.factor =
      age %>%
      cut(breaks = c(4,20,40,60,95), include.lowest = TRUE) %>%
      fct_recode(
        "≤20"      = "[4,20]",
        "21 to 40" = "(20,40]",
        "41 to 60" = "(40,60]",
        ">60"      = "(60,95]"
      ) %>%
      ff_label("Age (years)")
  )
head(meldata$age.factor)
```

```
## [1] >60       41 to 60 41 to 60 >60      41 to 60 21 to 40
## Levels: ≤20 21 to 40 41 to 60 >60
```

8.7　Plot the data

We are interested in the association between tumour ulceration and death from melanoma. To start then, we simply count the number of patients with ulcerated tumours who died. It is useful to plot this as counts but also as proportions. It is proportions you are comparing, but you really want to know the absolute numbers as well.

```
p1 <- meldata %>%
  ggplot(aes(x = ulcer.factor, fill = status.factor)) +
  geom_bar() +
  theme(legend.position = "none")

p2 <- meldata %>%
  ggplot(aes(x = ulcer.factor, fill = status.factor)) +
  geom_bar(position = "fill") +
  ylab("proportion")

library(patchwork)
p1 + p2
```

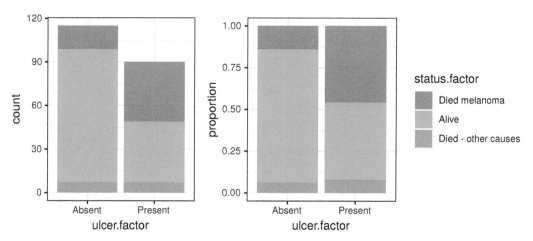

FIGURE 8.2: Bar chart: Outcome after surgery for patients with ulcerated melanoma.

It should be obvious that more died from melanoma in the ulcerated tumour group compared with the non-ulcerated tumour group. The stacking is orders from top to bottom by default. This can be easily adjusted by changing the order of the levels within the factor (see re-levelling below). This default order works well for binary variables - the "yes" or "1" is lowest and can be easily compared. This ordering of this particular variable is unusual - it would be more common to have for instance `alive = 0`, `died = 1`. One quick option is to just reverse the order of the levels in the plot.

```
p1 <- meldata %>%
  ggplot(aes(x = ulcer.factor, fill = status.factor)) +
  geom_bar(position = position_stack(reverse = TRUE)) +
  theme(legend.position = "none")

p2 <- meldata %>%
  ggplot(aes(x = ulcer.factor, fill = status.factor)) +
  geom_bar(position = position_fill(reverse = TRUE)) +
  ylab("proportion")

library(patchwork)
p1 + p2
```

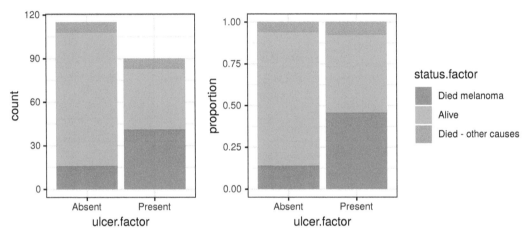

FIGURE 8.3: Bar chart: Outcome after surgery for patients with ulcerated melanoma, reversed levels.

Just from the plot then, death from melanoma in the ulcerated tumour group is around 40% and in the non-ulcerated group around 13%. The number of patients included in the study is not huge, however, this still looks like a real difference given its effect size.

We may also be interested in exploring potential effect modification, interactions and confounders. Again, we urge you to first visualise these, rather than going straight to a model.

```
p1 <- meldata %>%
  ggplot(aes(x = ulcer.factor, fill=status.factor)) +
  geom_bar(position = position_stack(reverse = TRUE)) +
  facet_grid(sex.factor ~ age.factor) +
  theme(legend.position = "none")

p2 <- meldata %>%
  ggplot(aes(x = ulcer.factor, fill=status.factor)) +
  geom_bar(position = position_fill(reverse = TRUE)) +
  facet_grid(sex.factor ~ age.factor)+
  theme(legend.position = "bottom")
```

p1 / p2

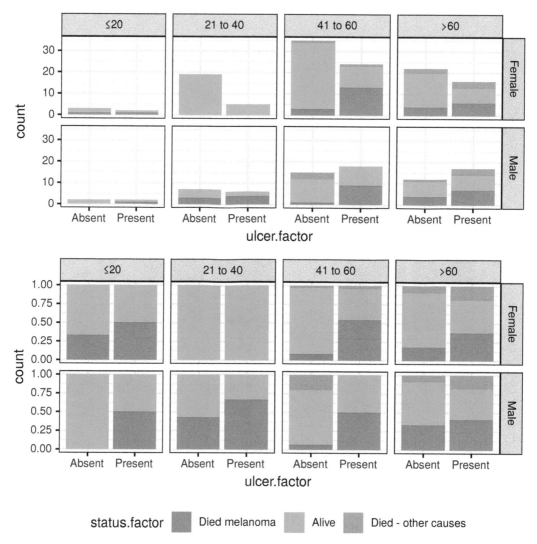

FIGURE 8.4: Facetted bar plot: Outcome after surgery for patients with ulcerated melanoma aggregated by sex and age.

8.8 Group factor levels together - `fct_collapse()`

Our question relates to the association between tumour ulceration and death from melanoma. The outcome measure has three levels as can be seen. For our purposes here, we will generate a disease-specific mortality variable (`status_dss`), by combining "Died - other causes" and "Alive".

```
meldata <- meldata %>%
  mutate(
    status_dss = fct_collapse(
      status.factor,
      "Alive" = c("Alive", "Died - other causes"))
  )
```

8.9 Change the order of values within a factor - `fct_relevel()`

The default order for levels with `factor()` is alphabetical. We often want to reorder the levels in a factor when plotting, or when performing a regression analysis and we want to specify the reference level.

The order can be checked using `levels()`.

```
# dss - disease specific survival
meldata$status_dss %>% levels()
```

```
## [1] "Died melanoma" "Alive"
```

The reason "Alive" is second, rather than alphabetical, is it was recoded from "2" and that order was retained. If, however, we want to make comparisons relative to "Alive", we need to move it to the front by using `fct_relevel()`.

```
meldata <- meldata %>%
  mutate(status_dss = status_dss %>%
           fct_relevel("Alive")
         )
```

Any number of factor levels can be specified in `fct_relevel()`.

8.10 Summarising factors with `finalfit`

Our own **finalfit** package provides convenient functions to summarise and compare factors, producing final tables for publication.

```
library(finalfit)
meldata %>%
  summary_factorlist(dependent   = "status_dss",
                explanatory = "ulcer.factor")
```

TABLE 8.1: Two-by-two table with finalfit: Died with melanoma by tumour ulceration status.

label	levels		Alive	Died melanoma
Ulcerated tumour	Absent	99 (66.9)	16 (28.1)
	Present	49 (33.1)	41 (71.9)

finalfit is useful for summarising multiple variables. We often want to summarise more than one factor or continuous variable against our dependent variable of interest. Think of Table 1 in a journal article.

Any number of continuous or categorical explanatory variables can be added.

```
library(finalfit)
meldata %>%
  summary_factorlist(dependent = "status_dss",
                explanatory =
                    c("ulcer.factor", "age.factor",
                      "sex.factor", "thickness")
  )
```

TABLE 8.2: Multiple variables by outcome: Outcome after surgery for melanoma by patient and disease factors.

label	levels	Alive	Died melanoma
Ulcerated tumour	Absent	99 (66.9)	16 (28.1)
	Present	49 (33.1)	41 (71.9)
Age (years)	20	6 (4.1)	3 (5.3)
	21 to 40	30 (20.3)	7 (12.3)
	41 to 60	66 (44.6)	26 (45.6)
	>60	46 (31.1)	21 (36.8)
Sex	Female	98 (66.2)	28 (49.1)
	Male	50 (33.8)	29 (50.9)
thickness	Mean (SD)	2.4 (2.5)	4.3 (3.6)

8.11 Pearson's chi-squared and Fisher's exact tests

Pearson's chi-squared (χ^2) test of independence is used to determine whether two categorical variables are independent in a given population. Independence here means that the relative frequencies of one variable are the same over all levels of another variable.

A common setting for this is the classic 2x2 table. This refers to two categorical variables with exactly two levels each, such as is show in Table 8.1 above. The null hypothesis of independence for this particular question is no difference in the proportion of patients with ulcerated tumours who die (45.6%) compared with non-ulcerated tumours (13.9%). From the raw frequencies, there seems to be a large difference, as we noted in the plot we made above.

8.11.1 Base R

Base R has reliable functions for all common statistical tests, but they are sometimes a little inconvenient to extract results from.

A table of counts can be constructed, either using the $ to identify columns, or using the `with()` function.

```
table(meldata$ulcer.factor, meldata$status_dss) # both give same result
with(meldata, table(ulcer.factor, status_dss))
```

```
##
##            Alive Died melanoma
##   Absent     99           16
##   Present    49           41
```

When working with older R functions, a useful shortcut is the exposition pipe-operator (`%$%`) from the **magrittr** package, home of the standard forward pipe-operator (`%>%`). The exposition pipe-operator exposes data frame/tibble columns on the left to the function which follows on the right. It's easier to see in action by making a table of counts.

```
library(magrittr)
meldata %$%            # note $ sign here
  table(ulcer.factor, status_dss)
```

```
##              status_dss
## ulcer.factor Alive Died melanoma
##      Absent     99           16
##      Present    49           41
```

The counts table can be passed to `prop.table()` for proportions.

```
meldata %$%
  table(ulcer.factor, status_dss) %>%
  prop.table(margin = 1)     # 1: row, 2: column etc.
```

```
##              status_dss
## ulcer.factor    Alive Died melanoma
##       Absent 0.8608696        0.1391304
##       Present 0.5444444       0.4555556
```

Similarly, the counts table can be passed to `chisq.test()` to perform the chi-squared test.

```
meldata %$%          # note $ sign here
  table(ulcer.factor, status_dss) %>%
  chisq.test()
```

```
##
##  Pearson's Chi-squared test with Yates' continuity correction
##
## data:  .
## X-squared = 23.631, df = 1, p-value = 1.167e-06
```

The result can be extracted into a tibble using the `tidy()` function from the **broom** package.

```
library(broom)
meldata %$%          # note $ sign here
  table(ulcer.factor, status_dss) %>%
  chisq.test() %>%
  tidy()
```

```
## # A tibble: 1 x 4
##   statistic   p.value parameter method
##       <dbl>     <dbl>     <int> <chr>
## 1      23.6 0.00000117         1 Pearson's Chi-squared test with Yates' continu~
```

The `chisq.test()` function applies the Yates' continuity correction by default. The standard interpretation assumes that the discrete probability of observed counts in the table can be approximated by the continuous chi-squared distribution. This introduces some error. The correction involves subtracting 0.5 from the absolute difference between each observed and expected value. This is particularly helpful when counts are low, but can be removed if desired by `chisq.test(..., correct = FALSE)`.

8.12 Fisher's exact test

A commonly stated assumption of the chi-squared test is the requirement to have an expected count of at least 5 in each cell of the 2x2 table. For larger tables, all expected counts should be > 1 and no more than 20% of all cells should have expected counts < 5. If this assumption is not fulfilled, an alternative test is Fisher's exact test. For instance, if we are testing across a 2x4 table created from our `age.factor` variable and `status_dss`, then we receive a warning.

```
meldata %$%           # note $ sign here
  table(age.factor, status_dss) %>%
  chisq.test()
```

```
## Warning in chisq.test(.): Chi-squared approximation may be incorrect

##
##   Pearson's Chi-squared test
##
## data:  .
## X-squared = 2.0198, df = 3, p-value = 0.5683
```

Switch to Fisher's exact test

```
meldata %$%           # note $ sign here
  table(age.factor, status_dss) %>%
  fisher.test()
```

```
##
##   Fisher's Exact Test for Count Data
##
## data:  .
## p-value = 0.5437
## alternative hypothesis: two.sided
```

8.13 Chi-squared / Fisher's exact test using finalfit

It is easier using the `summary_factorlist()` function from the **finalfit** package. Including `p = TRUE` in `summary_factorlist()` adds a hypothesis test to each included comparison. This defaults to chi-squared tests with a continuity correction for categorical variables.

```
library(finalfit)
meldata %>%
  summary_factorlist(dependent   = "status_dss",
                     explanatory = "ulcer.factor",
                     p = TRUE)
```

TABLE 8.3: Two-by-two table with chi-squared test using final fit: Outcome after surgery for melanoma by tumour ulceration status.

label	levels	Alive	Died melanoma	p
Ulcerated tumour	Absent	99 (66.9)	16 (28.1)	<0.001
	Present	49 (33.1)	41 (71.9)	

Adding further variables:

```
meldata %>%
  summary_factorlist(dependent = "status_dss",
                     explanatory =
                       c("ulcer.factor", "age.factor",
                         "sex.factor", "thickness"),
                     p = TRUE)
```

```
## Warning in chisq.test(age.factor, status_dss): Chi-squared approximation may be
## incorrect
```

TABLE 8.4: Multiple variables by outcome with hypothesis tests: Outcome after surgery for melanoma by patient and disease factors (chi-squared test).

label	levels	Alive	Died melanoma	p
Ulcerated tumour	Absent	99 (66.9)	16 (28.1)	<0.001
	Present	49 (33.1)	41 (71.9)	
Age (years)	20	6 (4.1)	3 (5.3)	0.568
	21 to 40	30 (20.3)	7 (12.3)	
	41 to 60	66 (44.6)	26 (45.6)	
	>60	46 (31.1)	21 (36.8)	
Sex	Female	98 (66.2)	28 (49.1)	0.036
	Male	50 (33.8)	29 (50.9)	
thickness	Mean (SD)	2.4 (2.5)	4.3 (3.6)	<0.001

Note that for continuous expanatory variables, an F-test (ANOVA) is performed by default. If variables are considered non-parametric (cont = "mean"), then a Kruskal-Wallis test is used.

Switch to Fisher's exact test:

```
meldata %>%
  summary_factorlist(dependent = "status_dss",
                    explanatory =
                      c("ulcer.factor", "age.factor",
                        "sex.factor", "thickness"),
                    p = TRUE,
                    p_cat = "fisher")
```

TABLE 8.5: Multiple variables by outcome with hypothesis tests: Outcome after surgery for melanoma by patient and disease factors (Fisher's exact test).

label	levels	Alive	Died melanoma	p
Ulcerated tumour	Absent	99 (66.9)	16 (28.1)	<0.001
	Present	49 (33.1)	41 (71.9)	
Age (years)	20	6 (4.1)	3 (5.3)	0.544
	21 to 40	30 (20.3)	7 (12.3)	
	41 to 60	66 (44.6)	26 (45.6)	
	>60	46 (31.1)	21 (36.8)	
Sex	Female	98 (66.2)	28 (49.1)	0.026
	Male	50 (33.8)	29 (50.9)	
thickness	Mean (SD)	2.4 (2.5)	4.3 (3.6)	<0.001

Further options can be included:

```
meldata %>%
  summary_factorlist(dependent = "status_dss",
                    explanatory =
                      c("ulcer.factor", "age.factor",
                        "sex.factor", "thickness"),
                    p = TRUE,
                    p_cat = "fisher",
                    digits =
                      c(1, 1, 4, 2), #1: mean/median, 2: SD/IQR
                                     # 3: p-value, 4: count percentage
                    na_include = TRUE, # include missing in results/test
                    add_dependent_label = TRUE
  )
```

TABLE 8.6: Multiple variables by outcome with hypothesis tests: Options including missing data, rounding, and labels.

Dependent: Status		Alive	Died melanoma	p
Ulcerated tumour	Absent	99 (66.89)	16 (28.07)	<0.0001
	Present	49 (33.11)	41 (71.93)	
Age (years)	20	6 (4.05)	3 (5.26)	0.5437
	21 to 40	30 (20.27)	7 (12.28)	
	41 to 60	66 (44.59)	26 (45.61)	
	>60	46 (31.08)	21 (36.84)	
Sex	Female	98 (66.22)	28 (49.12)	0.0263
	Male	50 (33.78)	29 (50.88)	
thickness	Mean (SD)	2.4 (2.5)	4.3 (3.6)	<0.0001

8.14 Exercises

8.14.1 Exercise

Using `finalfit`, create a summary table with "status.factor" as the dependent variable and the following as explanatory variables: `sex.factor`, `ulcer.factor`, `age.factor`, `thickness`.

Change the continuous variable summary statistic to `median` and `interquartile range` instead of `mean` and `sd`.

8.14.2 Exercise

By changing one and only one line in the following block create firstly a new table showing the breakdown of `status.factor` by age and secondly the breakdown of `status.factor` by sex:

```
meldata %>%
  count(ulcer.factor, status.factor) %>%
  group_by(status.factor) %>%
  mutate(total = sum(n)) %>%
  mutate(percentage = round(100*n/total, 1)) %>%
  mutate(count_perc = paste0(n, " (", percentage, ")")) %>%
  select(-total, -n, -percentage) %>%
  spread(status.factor, count_perc)
```

8.14.3 Exercise

Now produce these tables using the `summary_factorlist()` function from the **finalfit** package.

9

Logistic regression

All generalizations are false, including this one.
Mark Twain

9.1 Generalised linear modelling

Do not start here! The material covered in this chapter is best understood after having read linear regression (Chapter 7) and working with categorical outcome variables (Chapter 8).

Generalised linear modelling is an extension to the linear modelling we are now familiar with. It allows the principles of linear regression to be applied when outcomes are not continuous numeric variables.

9.2 Binary logistic regression

A regression analysis is a statistical approach to estimating the relationships between variables, often by drawing straight lines through data points. For instance, we may try to predict blood pressure in a group of patients based on their coffee consumption (Figure 7.1 from Chapter 7). As blood pressure and coffee consumption can be considered on a continuous scale, this is an example of simple linear regression.

Logistic regression is an extension of this, where the variable being predicted is *categorical*. We will focus on binary logistic regression, where the dependent variable has two levels, e.g., yes or no, 0 or 1, dead or alive. Other types of logistic regression include 'ordinal', when the outcome variable has >2 ordered levels, and 'multinomial', where the outcome variable has >2 levels with no inherent order.

We will only deal with binary logistic regression. When we use the term 'logistic regression', that is what we are referring to.

We have good reason. In healthcare we are often interested in an event (like death) occurring or not occurring. Binary logistic regression can tell us the probability of this outcome occurring in a patient with a particular set of characteristics.

Although in binary logistic regression the outcome must have two levels, remember that the predictors (explanatory variables) can be either continuous or categorical.

9.2.1   The Question (1)

As in previous chapters, we will use concrete examples when discussing the principles of the approach. We return to our example of coffee drinking. Yes, we are a little obsessed with coffee.

Our outcome variable was previously blood pressure. We will now consider our outcome as the occurrence of a cardiovascular (CV) event over a 10-year period. A cardiovascular event includes the diagnosis of ischemic heart disease, a heart attack (myocardial infarction), or a stroke (cerebrovascular accident). The diagnosis of a cardiovascular event is clearly a binary condition, it either happens or it does not. This is ideal for modelling using binary logistic regression. But remember, the data are completely simulated and not based on anything in the real world. This bit is just for fun!

9.2.2   Odds and probabilities

To understand logistic regression we need to remind ourselves about odds and probability. Odds and probabilities can get confusing so get them straight with Figure 9.1.

In many situations, there is no particular reason to prefer one to the other. However, humans seem to have a preference for expressing chance in terms of probabilities, while odds have particular mathematical properties that make them useful in regression.

When a probability is 0, the odds are 0. When a probability is between 0 and 0.5, the odds are less than 1.0 (i.e., less than "1 to 1"). As probability increases from 0.5 to 1.0, the odds increase from 1.0 to approach infinity.

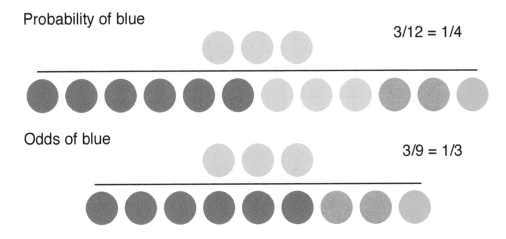

FIGURE 9.1: Probability vs odds.

Thus the range of probability is 0 to 1 and the range of odds is 0 to $+\infty$.

Odds and probabilities can easily be interconverted. For example, if the odds of a patient dying from a disease are 1/3 (in horse racing this is stated as '3 to 1 against'), then the probability of death (also known as risk) is 0.25 (or 25%). Odds of 1 to 1 equal 50%.

$Odds = \frac{p}{1-p}$, where p is the probability of the outcome occurring.

$Probability = \frac{odds}{odds+1}$.

9.2.3 Odds ratios

Another important term to remind ourselves of is the 'odds ratio'. Why? Because in a logistic regression the slopes of fitted lines (coefficients) can be interpreted as odds ratios. This is very useful when interpreting the association of a particular predictor with an outcome.

For a given categorical predictor such as smoking, the difference in chance of the outcome occurring for smokers vs non-smokers can be expressed as a ratio of odds or odds ratio (Figure 9.2). For example, if the odds of a smoker having a CV event are 1.5 and the odds of a non-smoker are 1.0, then the odds of a smoker having an event are 1.5-times greater than a non-smoker, odds ratio = 1.5.

An alternative is a ratio of probabilities which is called a risk ratio or relative risk. We will continue to work with odds ratios given they are an important expression of effect size in logistic regression analysis.

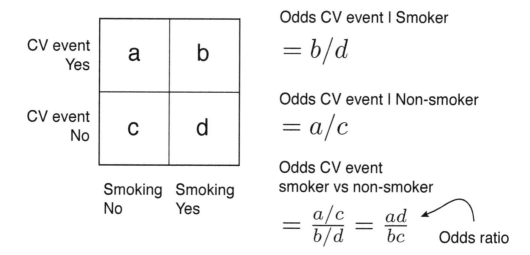

FIGURE 9.2: Odds ratios.

9.2.4 Fitting a regression line

Let's return to the task at hand. The difficulty in moving from a continuous to a binary outcome variable quickly becomes obvious. If our y-axis only has two values, say 0 and 1, then how can we fit a line through our data points?

An assumption of linear regression is that the dependent variable is continuous, unbounded, and measured on an interval or ratio scale. Unfortunately, binary dependent variables fulfil none of these requirements.

The answer is what makes logistic regression so useful. Rather than estimating $y = 0$ or $y = 1$ from the x-axis, we estimate the *probability* of $y = 1$.

There is one more difficulty in this though. Probabilities can only exist for values of 0 to 1. The probability scale is therefore not linear - straight lines do not make sense on it.

As we saw above, the odds scale runs from 0 to $+\infty$. But here, probabilities from 0 to 0.5 are squashed into odds of 0 to 1, and probabilities from 0.5 to 1 have the expansive comfort of 1 to $+\infty$.

This is why we fit binary data on a *log-odds scale*.

A log-odds scale sounds incredibly off-putting to non-mathematicians, but it is the perfect solution.

- Log-odds run from $-\infty$ to $+\infty$;
- odds of 1 become log-odds of 0;
- a doubling and a halving of odds represent the same distance on the scale.

```
log(1)
```

```
## [1] 0
```

```
log(2)
```

```
## [1] 0.6931472
```

```
log(0.5)
```

```
## [1] -0.6931472
```

I'm sure some are shouting 'obviously' at the page. That is good!

This is wrapped up in a transformation (a bit like the transformations shown in Section 6.9.1) using the so-called logit function. This can be skipped with no loss of understanding, but for those who just-gots-to-see, the logit function is,

$\log_e(\frac{p}{1-p})$, where p is the probability of the outcome occurring.

Figure 9.3 demonstrates the fitted lines from a logistic regression model of cardiovascular event by coffee consumption, stratified by smoking on the log-odds scale (A) and the probability scale (B). We could conclude, for instance, that on average, non-smokers who drink 2 cups of coffee per day have a 50% chance of a cardiovascular event.

9.2.5   The fitted line and the logistic regression equation

Figure 9.4 links the logistic regression equation, the appearance of the fitted lines on the probability scale, and the output from a standard base R analysis. The dots at the top and bottom of the plot represent whether individual patients have had an event or not. The fitted line, therefore, represents the point-to-point probability of a patient with a particular set of characteristics having the event or not. Compare this to Figure 7.4 to be clear on the difference. The slope of the line is linear on the log-odds scale and these are presented in the output on the log-odds scale.

Thankfully, it is straightforward to convert these to odds ratios, a measure we can use to communicate effect size and direction effectively. Said in more technical language, the exponential of the coefficient on the log-odds scale can be interpreted as an odds ratio.

For a continuous variable such as cups of coffee consumed, the odds ratio is the change in odds of a CV event associated with a 1 cup increase in coffee

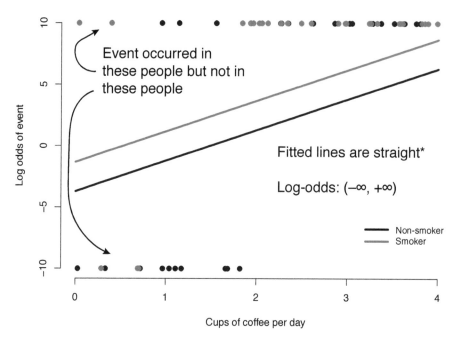

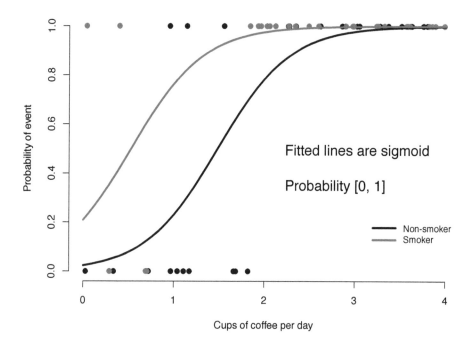

FIGURE 9.3: A logistic regression model of life-time cardiovascular event occurrence by coffee consumption stratified by smoking (simulated data). Fitted lines plotted on the log-odds scale (A) and probability scale (B). *lines are straight when no polynomials or splines are included in regression.

consumption. We are dealing with linear responses here, so the odds ratio is the same for an increase from 1 to 2 cups, or 3 to 4 cups etc. Remember that if the odds ratio for 1 unit of change is 1.5, then the odds ratio for 2 units of change is $exp(log(1.5) * 2) = 2.25$.

For a categorical variable such as smoking, the odds ratio is the change in odds of a CV event associated with smoking compared with not smoking (the reference level).

9.2.6 Effect modification and confounding

As with all multivariable regression models, logistic regression allows the incorporation of multiple variables which all may have direct effects on outcome or may confound the effect of another variable. This was explored in detail in Section 7.1.7; all of the same principles apply.

Adjusting for effect modification and confounding allows us to isolate the direct effect of an explanatory variable of interest upon an outcome. In our example, we are interested in direct effect of coffee drinking on the occurrence of cardiovascular disease, independent of any association between coffee drinking and smoking.

Figure 9.5 demonstrates simple, additive and multiplicative models. Think back to Figure 7.6 and the discussion around it as these terms are easier to think about when looking at the linear regression example, but essentially they work the same way in logistic regression.

Presented on the probability scale, the effect of the interaction is difficult to see. It is obvious on the log-odds scale that the fitted lines are no longer constrained to be parallel.

The interpretation of the interaction term is important. The exponential of the interaction coefficient term represents a 'ratio-of-odds ratios'. This is easiest to see through a worked example. In Figure 9.6 the effect of coffee on the odds of a cardiovascular event can be compared in smokers and non-smokers. The effect is now different given the inclusion of a significant interaction term. Please check back to the linear regression chapter if this is not making sense.

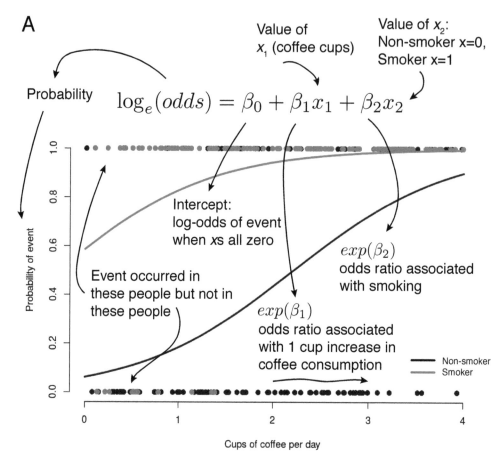

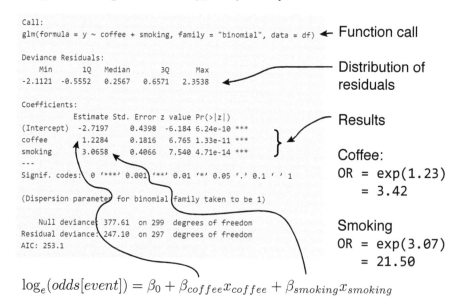

FIGURE 9.4: Linking the logistic regression fitted line and equation (A) with the R output (B).

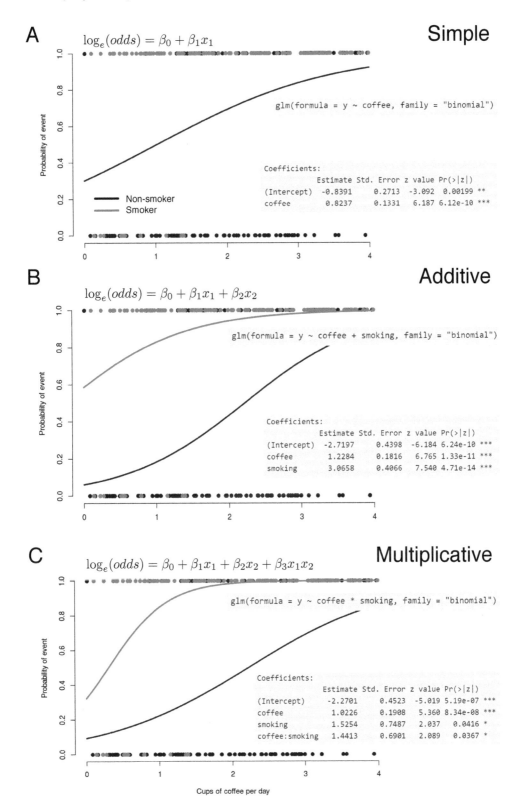

FIGURE 9.5: Multivariable logistic regression (A) with additive (B) and multiplicative (C) effect modification.

Multiplicative / interaction model

$$\log_e(odds) = \beta_0 + \beta_1 x_1 + \beta_2 x_2 + \beta_3 x_1 x_2$$ `glm(formula = y ~ coffee * smoking, family = "binomial")`

```
Coefficients:
                Estimate Std. Error z value Pr(>|z|)
(Intercept)     -2.2701     0.4523   -5.019 5.19e-07 ***
coffee           1.0226     0.1908    5.360 8.34e-08 ***
smoking          1.5254     0.7487    2.037   0.0416 *
coffee:smoking   1.4413     0.6901    2.089   0.0367 *
```

OR = exp(1.0226) = 2.78
OR = exp(1.5254) = 4.60
ROR = exp(1.4413) = 4.23

	Odds ratio (OR)
Effect of each coffee in non-smokers	2.78
Effect of each coffee in smokers	(2.78 * 4.23) = 11.76
Effect of smoking in non-coffee drinkers	OR = 4.60
Effect of smoking for each additional coffee	(4.60 * 4.23) = 19.46

FIGURE 9.6: Multivariable logistic regression with interaction term. The exponential of the interaction term is a ratio-of-odds ratios (ROR).

9.3   Data preparation and exploratory analysis

9.3.1   The Question (2)

We will go on to explore the `boot::melanoma` dataset introduced in Chapter 8. The data consist of measurements made on patients after surgery to remove the melanoma skin cancer in the University Hospital of Odense, Denmark, between 1962 and 1977.

Malignant melanoma is an aggressive and highly invasive cancer, making it difficult to treat.

To determine how advanced it is, staging is based on the depth of the tumour. The current TNM classification cut-offs are:

- T1: ≤ 1.0 mm depth
- T2: 1.1 to 2.0 mm depth
- T3: 2.1 to 4.0 mm depth
- T4: > 4.0 mm depth

This will be important in our analysis as we will create a new variable based upon this.

Using logistic regression, we will investigate factors associated with death from malignant melanoma with particular interest in tumour ulceration.

9.3.2 Get the data

The Help page (F1 on `boot::melanoma`) gives us its data dictionary including the definition of each variable and the coding used.

```
melanoma <- boot::melanoma
```

9.3.3 Check the data

As before, always carefully check and clean new dataset before you start the analysis.

```
library(tidyverse)
library(finalfit)
melanoma %>% glimpse()
melanoma %>% ff_glimpse()
```

9.3.4 Recode the data

We have seen some of this already (Section 8.5: Recode data), but for this particular analysis we will recode some further variables.

```
library(tidyverse)
library(finalfit)
melanoma <- melanoma %>%
  mutate(sex.factor = factor(sex) %>%
           fct_recode("Female" = "0",
                      "Male"   = "1") %>%
           ff_label("Sex"),

         ulcer.factor = factor(ulcer) %>%
           fct_recode("Present" = "1",
                      "Absent"  = "0") %>%
           ff_label("Ulcerated tumour"),

         age  = ff_label(age,  "Age (years)"),
         year = ff_label(year, "Year"),

         status.factor = factor(status) %>%
           fct_recode("Died melanoma"  = "1",
                      "Alive" = "2",
                      "Died - other" = "3") %>%
           fct_relevel("Alive") %>%
           ff_label("Status"),

         t_stage.factor =
           thickness %>%
           cut(breaks = c(0, 1.0, 2.0, 4.0,
```

```
                            max(thickness, na.rm=TRUE)),
                include.lowest = TRUE)
  )
```

Check the `cut()` function has worked:

```
melanoma$t_stage.factor %>% levels()
```

```
## [1] "[0,1]"    "(1,2]"    "(2,4]"    "(4,17.4]"
```

Recode for ease.

```
melanoma <- melanoma %>%
  mutate(
    t_stage.factor =
      fct_recode(t_stage.factor,
                 "T1" = "[0,1]",
                 "T2" = "(1,2]",
                 "T3" = "(2,4]",
                 "T4" = "(4,17.4]") %>%
      ff_label("T-stage")
  )
```

We will now consider our outcome variable. With a binary outcome and health data, we often have to make a decision as to *when* to determine if that variable has occurred or not. In the next chapter we will look at survival analysis where this requirement is not needed.

Our outcome of interest is death from melanoma, but we need to decide when to define this.

A quick histogram of `time` stratified by `status.factor` helps. We can see that most people who died from melanoma did so before 5 years (Figure 9.7). We can also see that the status most of those who did not die is known beyond 5 years.

```
library(ggplot2)
melanoma %>%
  ggplot(aes(x = time/365)) +
  geom_histogram() +
  facet_grid(. ~ status.factor)
```

```
## `stat_bin()` using `bins = 30`. Pick better value with `binwidth`.
```

Let's decide then to look at 5-year mortality from melanoma. The definition of this will be at 5 years after surgery, who had died from melanoma and who had not.

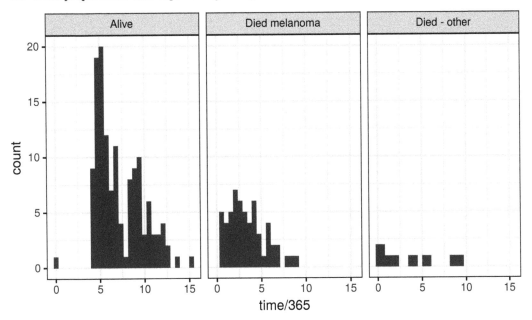

FIGURE 9.7: Time to outcome/follow-up times for patients in the melanoma dataset.

```
# 5-year mortality
melanoma <- melanoma %>%
  mutate(
    mort_5yr =
      if_else((time/365) < 5 &
                (status == 1),
              "Yes",              # then
              "No") %>%          # else
        fct_relevel("No") %>%
        ff_label("5-year survival")
  )
```

9.3.5 Plot the data

We are interested in the association between tumour ulceration and outcome (Figure 9.8).

```
p1 <- melanoma %>%
  ggplot(aes(x = ulcer.factor, fill = mort_5yr)) +
  geom_bar() +
  theme(legend.position = "none")

p2 <- melanoma %>%
  ggplot(aes(x = ulcer.factor, fill = mort_5yr)) +
  geom_bar(position = "fill") +
  ylab("proportion")
```

```
library(patchwork)
p1 + p2
```

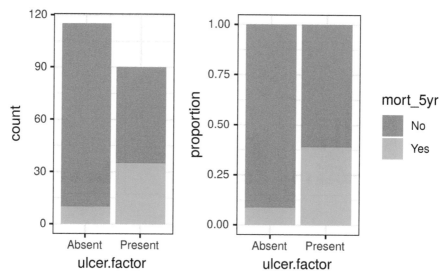

FIGURE 9.8: Exploration ulceration and outcome (5-year mortality).

As we might have anticipated from our work in the previous chapter, 5-year mortality is higher in patients with ulcerated tumours compared with those with non-ulcerated tumours.

We are also interested in other variables that may be associated with tumour ulceration. If they are also associated with our outcome, then they will confound the estimate of the direct effect of tumour ulceration.

We can plot out these relationships, or tabulate them instead.

9.3.6 Tabulate data

We will use the convenient `summary_factorlist()` function from the `finalfit` package to look for differences across other variables by tumour ulceration.

```
library(finalfit)
dependent <- "ulcer.factor"
explanatory <- c("age", "sex.factor", "year", "t_stage.factor")
melanoma %>%
  summary_factorlist(dependent, explanatory, p = TRUE,
                     add_dependent_label = TRUE)
```

It appears that patients with ulcerated tumours were older, more likely to

TABLE 9.1: Multiple variables by explanatory variable of interest: Malignant melanoma ulceration by patient and disease variables.

Dependent: Ulcerated tumour		Absent	Present	p
Age (years)	Mean (SD)	50.6 (15.9)	54.8 (17.4)	0.072
Sex	Female	79 (68.7)	47 (52.2)	0.024
	Male	36 (31.3)	43 (47.8)	
Year	Mean (SD)	1970.0 (2.7)	1969.8 (2.4)	0.637
T-stage	T1	51 (44.3)	5 (5.6)	<0.001
	T2	36 (31.3)	17 (18.9)	
	T3	21 (18.3)	30 (33.3)	
	T4	7 (6.1)	38 (42.2)	

be male, and had thicker/higher stage tumours. It is important therefore to consider inclusion of these variables in a regression model.

9.4 Model assumptions

Binary logistic regression is robust to many of the assumptions which cause problems in other statistical analyses. The main assumptions are:

1. Binary dependent variable - this is obvious, but as above we need to check (alive, death from disease, death from other causes doesn't work);
2. Independence of observations - the observations should not be repeated measurements or matched data;
3. Linearity of continuous explanatory variables and the log-odds outcome - take age as an example. If the outcome, say death, gets more frequent or less frequent as age rises, the model will work well. However, say children and the elderly are at high risk of death, but those in middle years are not, then the relationship is not linear. Or more correctly, it is not monotonic, meaning that the response does not only go in one direction;
4. No multicollinearity - explanatory variables should not be highly correlated with each other.

9.4.1 Linearity of continuous variables to the response

A graphical check of linearity can be performed using a best fit "loess" line. This is on the probability scale, so it is not going to be straight. But it should be monotonic - it should only ever go up or down.

```
melanoma %>%
  mutate(
    mort_5yr.num = as.numeric(mort_5yr) - 1
  ) %>%
  select(mort_5yr.num, age, year) %>%
  pivot_longer(all_of(c("age", "year")), names_to = "predictors") %>%
  ggplot(aes(x = value, y = mort_5yr.num)) +
  geom_point(size = 0.5, alpha = 0.5) +
  geom_smooth(method = "loess") +
  facet_wrap(~predictors, scales = "free_x")
```

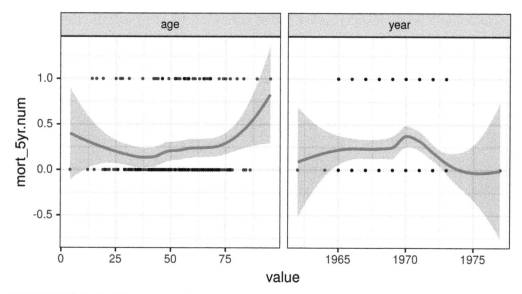

FIGURE 9.9: Linearity of our continuous explanatory variables to the outcome (5-year mortality).

Figure 9.9 shows that age is interesting as the relationship is u-shaped. The chance of death is higher in the young and the old compared with the middle-aged. This will need to be accounted for in any model including age as a predictor.

9.4.2 Multicollinearity

The presence of two or more highly correlated variables in a regression analysis can cause problems in the results which are generated. The slopes of lines (coefficients, ORs) can become unstable, which means big shifts in their size with minimal changes to the model or the underlying data. The confidence intervals around these coefficients may also be large. Definitions of the specifics differ between sources, but there are broadly two situations.

The first is when two highly correlated variables have been included in a model, sometimes referred to simply as collinearity. This can be detected by thinking about which variables may be correlated, and then checking using plotting.

The second situation is more devious. It is where collinearity exists between three or more variables, even when no pair of variables is particularly highly correlated. To detect this, we can use a specific metric called the *variance inflation factor*.

As always though, think clearly about your data and whether there may be duplication of information. Have you included a variable which is calculated from other variables already included in the model? Including body mass index (BMI), weight and height would be problematic, given the first is calculated from the latter two.

Are you describing a similar piece of information in two different ways? For instance, all perforated colon cancers are staged T4, so do you include T-stage and the perforation factor? (Note, not all T4 cancers have perforated.)

The `ggpairs()` function from `library(GGally)` is a good way of visualising all two-way associations (Figure 9.10).

```
library(GGally)
explanatory <- c("ulcer.factor", "age", "sex.factor",
                 "year", "t_stage.factor")
melanoma %>%
  remove_labels() %>%   # ggpairs doesn't work well with labels
  ggpairs(columns = explanatory)
```

If you have many variables you want to check you can split them up.

Continuous to continuous

Here we're using the same `library(GGally)` code as above, but shortlisting the two categorical variables: age and year (Figure 9.11):

```
select_explanatory <- c("age", "year")
melanoma %>%
  remove_labels() %>%
  ggpairs(columns = select_explanatory)
```

Continuous to categorical

Let's use a clever `pivot_longer()` and `facet_wrap()` combination to efficiently plot

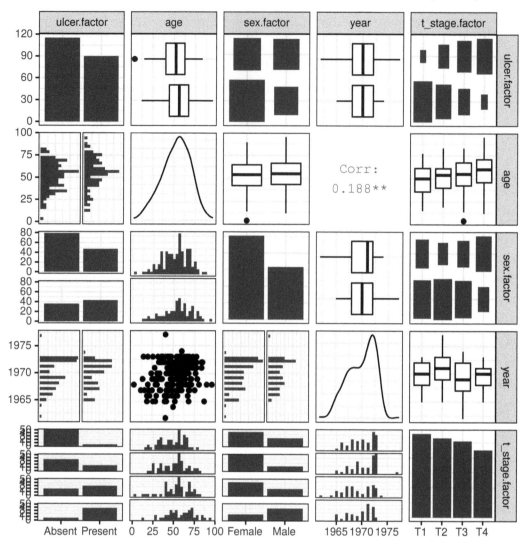

FIGURE 9.10: Exploring two-way associations within our explanatory variables.

multiple variables against each other without using `ggpairs()`. We want to compare everything against, for example, age so we need to include `-age` in the `pivot_longer()` call so it doesn't get lumped up with everything else (Figure 9.12):

```
select_explanatory <- c("age", "ulcer.factor",
                        "sex.factor", "t_stage.factor")

melanoma %>%
  select(all_of(select_explanatory)) %>%
  pivot_longer(-age) %>% # pivots all but age into two columns: name and value
  ggplot(aes(value, age)) +
  geom_boxplot() +
```

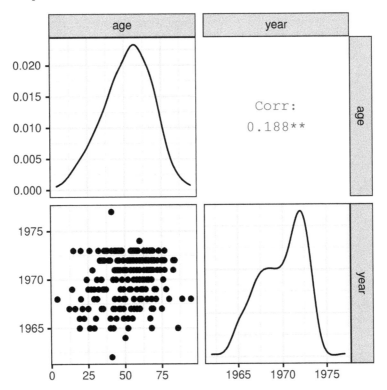

FIGURE 9.11: Exploring relationships between continuous variables.

```
facet_wrap(~name, scale = "free", ncol = 3) +
coord_flip()
```

Categorical to categorical

```
select_explanatory <- c("ulcer.factor", "sex.factor", "t_stage.factor")

melanoma %>%
  select(one_of(select_explanatory)) %>%
  pivot_longer(-sex.factor) %>%
  ggplot(aes(value, fill = sex.factor)) +
  geom_bar(position = "fill") +
  ylab("proportion") +
  facet_wrap(~name, scale = "free", ncol = 2) +
  coord_flip()
```

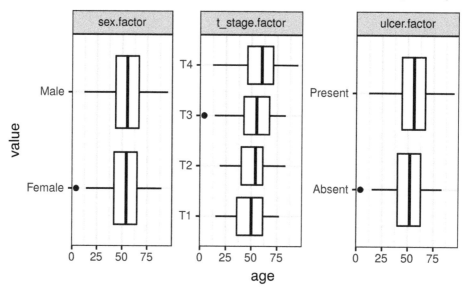

FIGURE 9.12: Exploring associations between continuous and categorical explanatory variables.

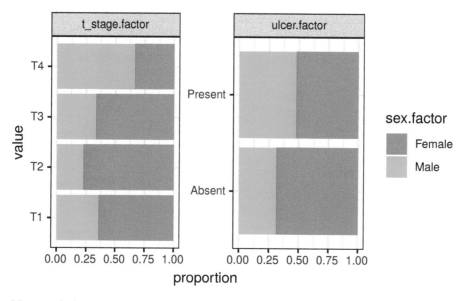

None of the explanatory variables are highly correlated with one another.

Variance inflation factor

Finally, as a final check for the presence of higher-order correlations, the variance inflation factor can be calculated for each of the terms in a final model. In simple language, this is a measure of how much the variance of a particular regression coefficient is increased due to the presence of multicollinearity in the model.

Here is an example. *GVIF* stands for generalised variance inflation factor. A common rule of thumb is that if this is greater than 5-10 for any variable, then multicollinearity may exist. The model should be further explored and the terms removed or reduced.

```
dependent <- "mort_5yr"
explanatory <- c("ulcer.factor", "age", "sex.factor",
                 "year", "t_stage.factor")
melanoma %>%
  glmmulti(dependent, explanatory) %>%
  car::vif()
```

```
##                     GVIF Df GVIF^(1/(2*Df))
## ulcer.factor    1.313355  1        1.146017
## age             1.102313  1        1.049911
## sex.factor      1.124990  1        1.060655
## year            1.102490  1        1.049995
## t_stage.factor  1.475550  3        1.066987
```

We are not trying to over-egg this, but multicollinearity can be important. The message as always is the same. Understand the underlying data using plotting and tables, and you are unlikely to come unstuck.

9.5 Fitting logistic regression models in base R

The glm() stands for generalised linear model and is the standard base R approach to logistic regression.

The glm() function has several options and many different types of model can be run. For instance, 'Poisson regression' for count data.

To run binary logistic regression use family = binomial. This defaults to family = binomial(link = 'logit'). Other link functions exist, such as the probit function, but this makes little difference to final conclusions.

Let's start with a simple univariable model using the classical R approach.

```
fit1 <- glm(mort_5yr ~ ulcer.factor, data = melanoma, family = binomial)
summary(fit1)
```

```
##
## Call:
## glm(formula = mort_5yr ~ ulcer.factor, family = binomial, data = melanoma)
##
## Deviance Residuals:
##     Min       1Q   Median       3Q      Max
## -0.9925  -0.9925  -0.4265  -0.4265   2.2101
##
```

```
## Coefficients:
##                      Estimate Std. Error z value Pr(>|z|)
## (Intercept)           -2.3514     0.3309  -7.105 1.20e-12 ***
## ulcer.factorPresent    1.8994     0.3953   4.805 1.55e-06 ***
## ---
## Signif. codes:  0 '***' 0.001 '**' 0.01 '*' 0.05 '.' 0.1 ' ' 1
##
## (Dispersion parameter for binomial family taken to be 1)
##
##     Null deviance: 215.78  on 204  degrees of freedom
## Residual deviance: 188.24  on 203  degrees of freedom
## AIC: 192.24
##
## Number of Fisher Scoring iterations: 5
```

This is the standard R output which you should become familiar with. It is included in the previous figures. The estimates of the coefficients (slopes) in this output are on the log-odds scale and always will be.

Easier approaches for doing this in practice are shown below, but for completeness here we will show how to extract the results. str() shows all the information included in the model object, which is useful for experts but a bit off-putting if you are starting out.

The coefficients and their 95% confidence intervals can be extracted and exponentiated like this.

```
coef(fit1) %>% exp()
```

```
##         (Intercept) ulcer.factorPresent
##           0.0952381           6.6818182
```

```
confint(fit1) %>% exp()
```

```
## Waiting for profiling to be done...
##                          2.5 %      97.5 %
## (Intercept)         0.04662675  0.1730265
## ulcer.factorPresent 3.18089978 15.1827225
```

Note that the 95% confidence interval is between the 2.5% and 97.5% quantiles of the distribution, hence why the results appear in this way.

A good alternative is the tidy() function from the **broom** package.

```
library(broom)
fit1 %>%
  tidy(conf.int = TRUE, exp = TRUE)
```

```
## # A tibble: 2 x 7
##   term          estimate std.error statistic  p.value conf.low conf.high
##   <chr>            <dbl>     <dbl>     <dbl>    <dbl>    <dbl>     <dbl>
```

```
## 1 (Intercept)            0.0952    0.331    -7.11 1.20e-12   0.0466    0.173
## 2 ulcer.factorPresent    6.68      0.395     4.80 1.55e- 6   3.18      15.2
```

We can see from these results that there is a strong association between tumour ulceration and 5-year mortality (OR 6.68, 95%CI 3.18, 15.18).

Model metrics can be extracted using the `glance()` function.

```
fit1 %>%
  glance()
```

```
## # A tibble: 1 x 8
##    null.deviance df.null logLik   AIC   BIC deviance df.residual  nobs
##            <dbl>   <int>  <dbl> <dbl> <dbl>    <dbl>       <int> <int>
## 1           216.     204  -94.1  192.  199.     188.         203   205
```

9.6 Modelling strategy for binary outcomes

A statistical model is a tool to understand the world. The better your model describes your data, the more useful it will be. Fitting a successful statistical model requires decisions around which variables to include in the model. Our advice regarding variable selection follows the same lines as in the linear regression chapter.

1. As few explanatory variables should be used as possible (parsimony);
2. Explanatory variables associated with the outcome variable in previous studies should be accounted for;
3. Demographic variables should be included in model exploration;
4. Population stratification should be incorporated if available;
5. Interactions should be checked and included if influential;
6. Final model selection should be performed using a "criterion-based approach"

- minimise the Akaike information criterion (AIC)
- maximise the c-statistic (area under the receiver operator curve).

We will use these principles through the next section.

9.7   Fitting logistic regression models with finalfit

Our preference in model fitting is now to use our own **finalfit** package. It gets us to our results quicker and more easily, and produces our final model tables which go directly into manuscripts for publication (we hope).

The approach is the same as in linear regression. If the outcome variable is correctly specified as a factor, the `finalfit()` function will run a logistic regression model directly.

```
library(finalfit)
dependent <- "mort_5yr"
explanatory <- "ulcer.factor"
melanoma %>%
  finalfit(dependent, explanatory, metrics = TRUE)
```

TABLE 9.2: Univariable logistic regression: 5-year survival from malignant melanoma by tumour ulceration (fit 1).

Dependent: 5-year survival		No	Yes	OR (univariable)	OR (multivariable)
Ulcerated tumour	Absent	105 (91.3)	10 (8.7)	-	-
	Present	55 (61.1)	35 (38.9)	6.68 (3.18-15.18, p<0.001)	6.68 (3.18-15.18, p<0.001)

TABLE 9.3: Model metrics: 5-year survival from malignant melanoma by tumour ulceration (fit 1).

Number in dataframe = 205, Number in model = 205, Missing = 0, AIC = 192.2, C-statistic = 0.717, H&L = Chi-sq(8) 0.00 (p=1.000)

9.7.1   Criterion-based model fitting

Passing `metrics = TRUE` to `finalfit()` gives us a useful list of model fitting parameters.

We recommend looking at three metrics:

- Akaike information criterion (AIC), which should be minimised,
- C-statistic (area under the receiver operator curve), which should be maximised;
- Hosmer–Lemeshow test, which should be non-significant.

AIC

The AIC has been previously described (Section 7.3.3). It provides a measure of model goodness-of-fit - or how well the model fits the available data. It is penalised for each additional variable, so should be somewhat robust against over-fitting (when the model starts to describe noise).

C-statistic

The c-statistic or area under the receiver operator curve (ROC) provides a measure of model 'discrimination'. It runs from 0.5 to 1.0, with 0.5 being no better than chance, and 1.0 being perfect fit. What the number actually represents can be thought of like this. Take our example of death from melanoma. If you take a random patient who died and a random patient who did not die, then the c-statistic is the probability that the model predicts that patient 1 is more likely to die than patient 2. In our example above, the model should get that correct 72% of the time.

Hosmer-Lemeshow test

If you are interested in using your model for prediction, it is important that it is calibrated correctly. Using our example, calibration means that the model accurately predicts death from melanoma when the risk to the patient is low and also accurately predicts death when the risk is high. The model should work well across the range of probabilities of death. The Hosmer-Lemeshow test assesses this. By default, it assesses the predictive accuracy for death in deciles of risk. If the model predicts equally well (or badly) at low probabilities compared with high probabilities, the null hypothesis of a difference will be rejected (meaning you get a non-significant p-value).

9.8 Model fitting

Engage with the data and the results when model fitting. Do not use automated processes - you have to keep thinking.

Three things are important to keep looking at:

- what is the association between a particular variable and the outcome (OR and 95%CI);
- how much information is a variable bringing to the model (change in AIC and c-statistic);
- how much influence does adding a variable have on the effect size of another variable, and in particular my variable of interest (a rule of thumb is seeing

a greater than 10% change in the OR of the variable of interest when a new variable is added to the model, suggests the new variable is important).

We're going to start by including the variables from above which we think are relevant.

```
library(finalfit)
dependent <- "mort_5yr"
explanatory <- c("ulcer.factor", "age", "sex.factor", "t_stage.factor")
fit2 = melanoma %>%
  finalfit(dependent, explanatory, metrics = TRUE)
```

TABLE 9.4: Multivariable logistic regression: 5-year survival from malignant melanoma (fit 2).

Dependent: 5-year survival		No	Yes	OR (univariable)	OR (multivariable)
Ulcerated tumour	Absent	105 (91.3)	10 (8.7)	-	-
	Present	55 (61.1)	35 (38.9)	6.68 (3.18-15.18, p<0.001)	3.21 (1.32-8.28, p=0.012)
Age (years)	Mean (SD)	51.7 (16.0)	55.3 (18.8)	1.01 (0.99-1.03, p=0.202)	1.00 (0.98-1.02, p=0.948)
Sex	Female	105 (83.3)	21 (16.7)	-	-
	Male	55 (69.6)	24 (30.4)	2.18 (1.12-4.30, p=0.023)	1.26 (0.57-2.76, p=0.558)
T-stage	T1	52 (92.9)	4 (7.1)	-	-
	T2	49 (92.5)	4 (7.5)	1.06 (0.24-4.71, p=0.936)	0.77 (0.16-3.58, p=0.733)
	T3	36 (70.6)	15 (29.4)	5.42 (1.80-20.22, p=0.005)	2.98 (0.86-12.10, p=0.098)
	T4	23 (51.1)	22 (48.9)	12.43 (4.21-46.26, p<0.001)	4.98 (1.34-21.64, p=0.021)

TABLE 9.5: Model metrics: 5-year survival from malignant melanoma (fit 2).

Number in dataframe = 205, Number in model = 205, Missing = 0, AIC = 188.1, C-statistic = 0.798, H&L = Chi-sq(8) 3.92 (p=0.864)

The model metrics have improved with the AIC decreasing from 192 to 188 and the c-statistic increasing from 0.717 to 0.798.

Let's consider age. We may expect age to be associated with the outcome because it so commonly is. But there is weak evidence of an association in the univariable analysis. We have shown above that the relationship of age to the outcome is not linear, therefore we need to act on this.

We can either convert age to a categorical variable or include it with a quadratic term ($x^2 + x$, remember parabolas from school?).

```
melanoma <- melanoma %>%
  mutate(
    age.factor = cut(age,
                     breaks = c(0, 25, 50, 75, 100)) %>%
    ff_label("Age (years)"))
```

```
# Add this to relevel:
# fct_relevel("(50,75]")

melanoma %>%
  finalfit(dependent, c("ulcer.factor", "age.factor"), metrics = TRUE)
```

TABLE 9.6: Multivariable logistic regression: using cut to convert a continuous variable as a factor (fit 3).

Dependent: 5-year survival		No	Yes	OR (univariable)	OR (multivariable)
Ulcerated tumour	Absent	105 (91.3)	10 (8.7)	-	-
	Present	55 (61.1)	35 (38.9)	6.68 (3.18-15.18, p<0.001)	6.28 (2.97-14.35, p<0.001)
Age (years)	(0,25]	10 (71.4)	4 (28.6)	-	-
	(25,50]	62 (84.9)	11 (15.1)	0.44 (0.12-1.84, p=0.229)	0.54 (0.13-2.44, p=0.400)
	(50,75]	79 (76.0)	25 (24.0)	0.79 (0.24-3.08, p=0.712)	0.81 (0.22-3.39, p=0.753)
	(75,100]	9 (64.3)	5 (35.7)	1.39 (0.28-7.23, p=0.686)	1.12 (0.20-6.53, p=0.894)

TABLE 9.7: Model metrics: using 'cut' to convert a continuous variable as a factor (fit 3).

Number in dataframe = 205, Number in model = 205, Missing = 0, AIC = 196.6, C-statistic = 0.742, H&L = Chi-sq(8) 0.20 (p=1.000)

There is no strong relationship between the categorical representation of age and the outcome. Let's try a quadratic term.

In base R, a quadratic term is added like this.

```
glm(mort_5yr ~ ulcer.factor  +I(age^2) + age,
    data = melanoma, family = binomial) %>%
  summary()
```

```
##
## Call:
## glm(formula = mort_5yr ~ ulcer.factor + I(age^2) + age, family = binomial,
##     data = melanoma)
##
## Deviance Residuals:
##     Min      1Q    Median      3Q      Max
## -1.3253  -0.8973  -0.4082  -0.3889   2.2872
##
## Coefficients:
##                       Estimate Std. Error z value Pr(>|z|)
## (Intercept)         -1.2636638  1.2058471  -1.048    0.295
## ulcer.factorPresent  1.8423431  0.3991559   4.616 3.92e-06 ***
## I(age^2)             0.0006277  0.0004613   1.361    0.174
## age                 -0.0567465  0.0476011  -1.192    0.233
## ---
## Signif. codes:  0 '***' 0.001 '**' 0.01 '*' 0.05 '.' 0.1 ' ' 1
##
```

```
## (Dispersion parameter for binomial family taken to be 1)
##
##       Null deviance: 215.78  on 204  degrees of freedom
## Residual deviance: 185.98  on 201  degrees of freedom
## AIC: 193.98
##
## Number of Fisher Scoring iterations: 5
```

It can be done in Finalfit in a similar manner. Note with default univariable model settings, the quadratic and linear terms are considered in separate models, which doesn't make much sense.

```
library(finalfit)
dependent <- "mort_5yr"
explanatory <- c("ulcer.factor", "I(age^2)", "age")
melanoma %>%
  finalfit(dependent, explanatory, metrics = TRUE)
```

TABLE 9.8: Multivariable logistic regression: including a quadratic term (fit 4).

Dependent: 5-year survival		No	Yes	OR (univariable)	OR (multivariable)
Ulcerated tumour	Absent	105 (91.3)	10 (8.7)	-	-
	Present	55 (61.1)	35 (38.9)	6.68 (3.18-15.18, p<0.001)	6.31 (2.98-14.44, p<0.001)
Age (years)	Mean (SD)	51.7 (16.0)	55.3 (18.8)	1.01 (0.99-1.03, p=0.202)	0.94 (0.86-1.04, p=0.233)
I(age^2)				1.00 (1.00-1.00, p=0.101)	1.00 (1.00-1.00, p=0.174)

TABLE 9.9: Model metrics: including a quadratic term (fit 4).

Number in dataframe = 205, Number in model = 205, Missing = 0, AIC = 194, C-statistic = 0.748, H&L = Chi-sq(8) 5.24 (p=0.732)

The AIC is worse when adding age either as a factor or with a quadratic term to the base model.

One final method to visualise the contribution of a particular variable is to remove it from the full model. This is convenient in Finalfit.

```
library(finalfit)
dependent <- "mort_5yr"
explanatory <- c("ulcer.factor", "age.factor", "sex.factor", "t_stage.factor")
explanatory_multi <- c("ulcer.factor", "sex.factor", "t_stage.factor")

melanoma %>%
  finalfit(dependent, explanatory, explanatory_multi,
           keep_models = TRUE, metrics = TRUE)
```

The AIC improves when age is removed (186 from 190) at only a small loss in discrimination (0.794 from 0.802). Looking at the model table and comparing

TABLE 9.10: Multivariable logistic regression model: comparing a reduced model in one table (fit 5).

Dependent: 5-year survival		No	Yes	OR (univariable)	OR (multivariable)	OR (multivariable reduced)
Ulcerated tumour	Absent	105 (91.3)	10 (8.7)	-	-	-
	Present	55 (61.1)	35 (38.9)	6.68 (3.18-15.18, p<0.001)	3.06 (1.25-7.93, p=0.017)	3.21 (1.32-8.28, p=0.012)
Age (years)	(0,25]	10 (71.4)	4 (28.6)	-	-	-
	(25,50]	62 (84.9)	11 (15.1)	0.44 (0.12-1.84, p=0.229)	0.37 (0.08-1.80, p=0.197)	-
	(50,75]	79 (76.0)	25 (24.0)	0.79 (0.24-3.08, p=0.712)	0.60 (0.15-2.65, p=0.469)	-
	(75,100]	9 (64.3)	5 (35.7)	1.39 (0.28-7.23, p=0.686)	0.61 (0.09-4.04, p=0.599)	-
Sex	Female	105 (83.3)	21 (16.7)	-	-	-
	Male	55 (69.6)	24 (30.4)	2.18 (1.12-4.30, p=0.023)	1.21 (0.54-2.68, p=0.633)	1.26 (0.57-2.76, p=0.559)
T-stage	T1	52 (92.9)	4 (7.1)	-	-	-
	T2	49 (92.5)	4 (7.5)	1.06 (0.24-4.71, p=0.936)	0.74 (0.15-3.50, p=0.697)	0.77 (0.16-3.58, p=0.733)
	T3	36 (70.6)	15 (29.4)	5.42 (1.80-20.22, p=0.005)	2.91 (0.84-11.82, p=0.106)	2.99 (0.86-12.11, p=0.097)
	T4	23 (51.1)	22 (48.9)	12.43 (4.21-46.26, p<0.001)	5.38 (1.43-23.52, p=0.016)	5.01 (1.37-21.52, p=0.020)

TABLE 9.11: Model metrics: comparing a reduced model in one table (fit 5).

Number in dataframe = 205, Number in model = 205, Missing = 0, AIC = 190, C-statistic = 0.802, H&L = Chi-sq(8) 13.87 (p=0.085)
Number in dataframe = 205, Number in model = 205, Missing = 0, AIC = 186.1, C-statistic = 0.794, H&L = Chi-sq(8) 1.07 (p=0.998)

the full multivariable with the reduced multivariable, there has been a small change in the OR for ulceration, with some of the variation accounted for by age now being taken up by ulceration. This is to be expected, given the association (albeit weak) that we saw earlier between age and ulceration. Given all this, we will decide not to include age in the model.

Now what about the variable sex. It has a significant association with the outcome in the univariable analysis, but much of this is explained by other variables in multivariable analysis. Is it contributing much to the model?

```
library(finalfit)
dependent <- "mort_5yr"
explanatory <- c("ulcer.factor", "sex.factor", "t_stage.factor")
explanatory_multi <- c("ulcer.factor", "t_stage.factor")

melanoma %>%
  finalfit(dependent, explanatory, explanatory_multi,
           keep_models = TRUE, metrics = TRUE)
```

By removing sex we have improved the AIC a little (184.4 from 186.1) with a small change in the c-statistic (0.791 from 0.794).

Looking at the model table, the variation has been taken up mostly by stage 4 disease and a little by ulceration. But there has been little change overall. We will exclude sex from our final model as well.

As a final we can check for a first-order interaction between ulceration and T-stage. Just to remind us what this means, a significant interaction would

TABLE 9.12: Multivariable logistic regression: further reducing the model (fit 6).

Dependent: 5-year survival		No	Yes	OR (univariable)	OR (multivariable)	OR (multivariable reduced)
Ulcerated tumour	Absent	105 (91.3)	10 (8.7)	-	-	-
	Present	55 (61.1)	35 (38.9)	6.68 (3.18-15.18, p<0.001)	3.21 (1.32-8.28, p=0.012)	3.26 (1.35-8.39, p=0.011)
Sex	Female	105 (83.3)	21 (16.7)	-	-	-
	Male	55 (69.6)	24 (30.4)	2.18 (1.12-4.30, p=0.023)	1.26 (0.57-2.76, p=0.559)	-
T-stage	T1	52 (92.9)	4 (7.1)	-	-	-
	T2	49 (92.5)	4 (7.5)	1.06 (0.24-4.71, p=0.936)	0.77 (0.16-3.58, p=0.733)	0.75 (0.16-3.45, p=0.700)
	T3	36 (70.6)	15 (29.4)	5.42 (1.80-20.22, p=0.005)	2.99 (0.86-12.11, p=0.097)	2.96 (0.86-11.96, p=0.098)
	T4	23 (51.1)	22 (48.9)	12.43 (4.21-46.26, p<0.001)	5.01 (1.37-21.52, p=0.020)	5.33 (1.48-22.56, p=0.014)

TABLE 9.13: Model metrics: further reducing the model (fit 6).

Number in dataframe = 205, Number in model = 205, Missing = 0, AIC = 186.1, C-statistic = 0.794, H&L = Chi-sq(8) 1.07 (p=0.998)
Number in dataframe = 205, Number in model = 205, Missing = 0, AIC = 184.4, C-statistic = 0.791, H&L = Chi-sq(8) 0.43 (p=1.000)

mean the effect of, say, ulceration on 5-year mortality would differ by T-stage. For instance, perhaps the presence of ulceration confers a much greater risk of death in advanced deep tumours compared with earlier superficial tumours.

```
library(finalfit)
dependent <- "mort_5yr"
explanatory <- c("ulcer.factor", "t_stage.factor")
explanatory_multi <- c("ulcer.factor*t_stage.factor")
melanoma %>%
   finalfit(dependent, explanatory, explanatory_multi,
        keep_models = TRUE, metrics = TRUE)
```

TABLE 9.14: Multivariable logistic regression: including an interaction term (fit 7).

label	levels	No	Yes	OR (univariable)	OR (multivariable)	OR (multivariable reduced)
Ulcerated tumour	Absent	105 (91.3)	10 (8.7)	-	-	-
	Present	55 (61.1)	35 (38.9)	6.68 (3.18-15.18, p<0.001)	3.26 (1.35-8.39, p=0.011)	4.00 (0.18-41.34, p=0.274)
T-stage	T1	52 (92.9)	4 (7.1)	-	-	-
	T2	49 (92.5)	4 (7.5)	1.06 (0.24-4.71, p=0.936)	0.75 (0.16-3.45, p=0.700)	0.94 (0.12-5.97, p=0.949)
	T3	36 (70.6)	15 (29.4)	5.42 (1.80-20.22, p=0.005)	2.96 (0.86-11.96, p=0.098)	3.76 (0.76-20.80, p=0.104)
	T4	23 (51.1)	22 (48.9)	12.43 (4.21-46.26, p<0.001)	5.33 (1.48-22.56, p=0.014)	2.67 (0.12-25.11, p=0.426)
UlcerPresent:T2	Interaction	-	-	-	-	0.57 (0.02-21.55, p=0.730)
UlcerPresent:T3	Interaction	-	-	-	-	0.62 (0.04-17.39, p=0.735)
UlcerPresent:T4	Interaction	-	-	-	-	1.85 (0.09-94.20, p=0.716)

There are no significant interaction terms.

Our final model table is therefore:

```
library(finalfit)
dependent <- "mort_5yr"
explanatory <- c("ulcer.factor", "age.factor",
            "sex.factor", "t_stage.factor")
```

```
explanatory_multi <- c("ulcer.factor", "t_stage.factor")
melanoma %>%
  finalfit(dependent, explanatory, explanatory_multi, metrics = TRUE)
```

TABLE 9.15: Multivariable logistic regression: final model (fit 8).

Dependent: 5-year survival		No	Yes	OR (univariable)	OR (multivariable)
Ulcerated tumour	Absent	105 (91.3)	10 (8.7)	-	-
	Present	55 (61.1)	35 (38.9)	6.68 (3.18-15.18, p<0.001)	3.26 (1.35-8.39, p=0.011)
Age (years)	(0,25]	10 (71.4)	4 (28.6)		-
	(25,50]	62 (84.9)	11 (15.1)	0.44 (0.12-1.84, p=0.229)	-
	(50,75]	79 (76.0)	25 (24.0)	0.79 (0.24-3.08, p=0.712)	-
	(75,100]	9 (64.3)	5 (35.7)	1.39 (0.28-7.23, p=0.686)	-
Sex	Female	105 (83.3)	21 (16.7)	-	-
	Male	55 (69.6)	24 (30.4)	2.18 (1.12-4.30, p=0.023)	-
T-stage	T1	52 (92.9)	4 (7.1)	-	-
	T2	49 (92.5)	4 (7.5)	1.06 (0.24-4.71, p=0.936)	0.75 (0.16-3.45, p=0.700)
	T3	36 (70.6)	15 (29.4)	5.42 (1.80-20.22, p=0.005)	2.96 (0.86-11.96, p=0.098)
	T4	23 (51.1)	22 (48.9)	12.43 (4.21-46.26, p<0.001)	5.33 (1.48-22.56, p=0.014)

TABLE 9.16: Model metrics: final model (fit 8).

Number in dataframe = 205, Number in model = 205, Missing = 0, AIC = 184.4, C-statistic = 0.791, H&L = Chi-sq(8) 0.43 (p=1.000)

9.8.1 Odds ratio plot

```
dependent <- "mort_5yr"
explanatory_multi <- c("ulcer.factor", "t_stage.factor")
melanoma %>%
  or_plot(dependent, explanatory_multi,
          breaks = c(0.5, 1, 2, 5, 10, 25),
          table_text_size = 3.5,
          title_text_size = 16)
```

```
## Warning: Removed 2 rows containing missing values (geom_errorbarh).
```

We can conclude that there is evidence of an association between tumour ulceration and 5-year survival which is independent of the tumour depth as captured by T-stage.

9.9 Correlated groups of observations

In our modelling strategy above, we mentioned the incorporation of population stratification if available. What does this mean?

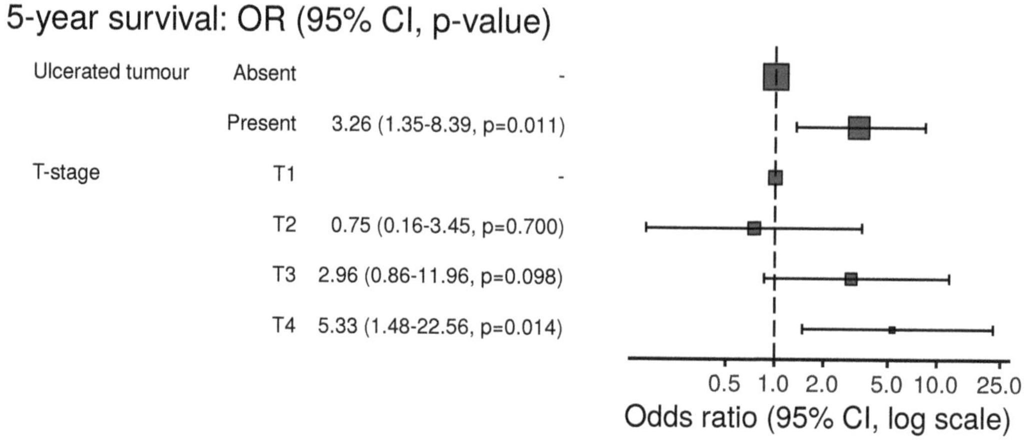

5-year survival: OR (95% CI, p-value)

Ulcerated tumour	Absent	-
	Present	3.26 (1.35-8.39, p=0.011)
T-stage	T1	-
	T2	0.75 (0.16-3.45, p=0.700)
	T3	2.96 (0.86-11.96, p=0.098)
	T4	5.33 (1.48-22.56, p=0.014)

0.5 1.0 2.0   5.0 10.0 25.0
Odds ratio (95% CI, log scale)

FIGURE 9.13: Odds ratio plot.

Our regression is seeking to capture the characteristics of particular patients. These characteristics are made manifest through the slopes of fitted lines - the estimated coefficients (ORs) of particular variables. A goal is to estimate these characteristics as precisely as possible. Bias can be introduced when correlations between patients are not accounted for. Correlations may be as simple as being treated within the same hospital. By virtue of this fact, these patients may have commonalities that have not been captured by the observed variables.

Population characteristics can be incorporated into our models. We may not be interested in capturing and measuring the effects themselves, but want to ensure they are accounted for in the analysis.

One approach is to include grouping variables as `random effects`. These may be nested with each other, for example patients within hospitals within countries. These are added in addition to the `fixed effects` we have been dealing with up until now.

These models go under different names including mixed effects model, multi-level model, or hierarchical model.

Other approaches, such as generalized estimating equations are not dealt with here.

9.9.1   Simulate data

Our melanoma dataset doesn't include any higher level structure, so we will simulate this for demonstration purposes. We have just randomly allocated 1 of 4 identifiers to each patient below.

```
# Simulate random hospital identifier
set.seed(1)
melanoma <- melanoma %>%
    mutate(hospital_id = sample(1:4, 205, replace = TRUE))

melanoma <- melanoma %>%
    mutate(hospital_id = c(rep(1:3, 50), rep(4, 55)))
```

9.9.2 Plot the data

We will speak in terms of 'hospitals' now, but the grouping variable(s) could clearly be anything.

The simplest random effects approach is a 'random intercept model'. This allows the intercept of fitted lines to vary by hospital. The random intercept model constrains lines to be parallel, in a similar way to the additive models discussed above and in Chapter 7.

It is harder to demonstrate with binomial data, but we can stratify the 5-year mortality by T-stage (considered as a continuous variable for this purpose). Note there were no deaths in 'hospital 4' (Figure 9.14). We can model this accounting for inter-hospital variation below.

```
melanoma %>%
    mutate(
    mort_5yr.num = as.numeric(mort_5yr) - 1 # Convert factor to 0 and 1
    ) %>%
    ggplot(aes(x = as.numeric(t_stage.factor), y = mort_5yr.num)) +
    geom_jitter(width = 0.1, height = 0.1) +
    geom_smooth(method = 'loess', se = FALSE) +
    facet_wrap(~hospital_id) +
    labs(x= "T-stage", y = "Mortality (5 y)")
```

```
## `geom_smooth()` using formula 'y ~ x'
```

9.9.3 Mixed effects models in base R

There are a number of different packages offering mixed effects modelling in R, our preferred is lme4.

```
library(lme4)
```

```
## Loading required package: Matrix
```

```
##
## Attaching package: 'Matrix'
```

```
## The following objects are masked from 'package:tidyr':
```

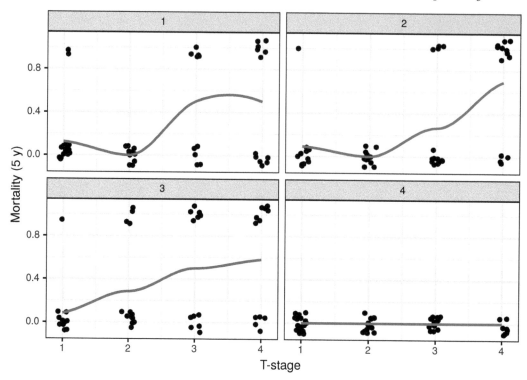

FIGURE 9.14: Investigating random effects by looking at the relationship between the outcome variable (5-year mortality) and T-stage at each hospital.

```
##
##      expand, pack, unpack

## Registered S3 methods overwritten by 'lme4':
##   method                           from
##   cooks.distance.influence.merMod  car
##   influence.merMod                 car
##   dfbeta.influence.merMod          car
##   dfbetas.influence.merMod         car


melanoma %>%
  glmer(mort_5yr ~ t_stage.factor + (1 | hospital_id),
        data = ., family = "binomial") %>%
  summary()


## Generalized linear mixed model fit by maximum likelihood (Laplace
##   Approximation) [glmerMod]
##  Family: binomial  ( logit )
## Formula: mort_5yr ~ t_stage.factor + (1 | hospital_id)
##    Data: .
##
##      AIC      BIC   logLik deviance df.resid
##    174.6    191.2    -82.3    164.6      200
##
## Scaled residuals:
##    Min      1Q  Median      3Q     Max
## -1.4507 -0.3930 -0.2891 -0.0640  3.4591
```

```
##
## Random effects:
##  Groups      Name         Variance Std.Dev.
##  hospital_id (Intercept) 2.619    1.618
## Number of obs: 205, groups:  hospital_id, 4
##
## Fixed effects:
##                   Estimate Std. Error z value Pr(>|z|)
## (Intercept)       -3.13132    1.01451  -3.087  0.00203 **
## t_stage.factorT2   0.02256    0.74792   0.030  0.97593
## t_stage.factorT3   1.82349    0.62920   2.898  0.00375 **
## t_stage.factorT4   2.61190    0.62806   4.159 3.2e-05 ***
## ---
## Signif. codes:  0 '***' 0.001 '**' 0.01 '*' 0.05 '.' 0.1 ' ' 1
##
## Correlation of Fixed Effects:
##            (Intr) t_s.T2 t_s.T3
## t_stg.fctT2 -0.365
## t_stg.fctT3 -0.454  0.591
## t_stg.fctT4 -0.459  0.590  0.718
```

The base R output is similar to `glm()`. It includes the standard deviation on the random effects intercept as well. Meaning the variation between hospitals being captured by the model.

The output can be examined using `tidy()` and `glance()` functions as above.

We find it more straightforward to use finalfit.

```
dependent <- "mort_5yr"
explanatory <- "t_stage.factor"
random_effect <- "hospital_id" # Is the same as:
random_effect <- "(1 | hospital_id)"
melanoma %>%
  finalfit(dependent, explanatory,
           random_effect = random_effect,
           metrics = TRUE)
```

We can incorporate our (made-up) hospital identifier into our final model from above. Using `keep_models = TRUE`, we can compare univariable, multivariable and mixed effects models.

```
library(finalfit)
dependent <- "mort_5yr"
explanatory <- c("ulcer.factor", "age.factor",
                 "sex.factor", "t_stage.factor")
explanatory_multi <- c("ulcer.factor", "t_stage.factor")
random_effect <- "hospital_id"
melanoma %>%
  finalfit(dependent, explanatory, explanatory_multi, random_effect,
           keep_models = TRUE,
           metrics = TRUE)
```

TABLE 9.17: Multilevel (mixed effects) logistic regression.

Dependent: 5-year survival		No	Yes	OR (univariable)	OR (multivariable)	OR (multivariable reduced)	OR (multilevel)
Ulcerated tumour	Absent	105 (91.3)	10 (8.7)	-	-	-	-
	Present	55 (61.1)	35 (38.9)	6.68 (3.18-15.18, p<0.001)	3.06 (1.25-7.93, p=0.017)	3.26 (1.35-8.39, p=0.011)	2.49 (0.94-6.59, p=0.065)
Age (years)	(0,25]	10 (71.4)	4 (28.6)	-	-	-	-
	(25,50]	62 (84.9)	11 (15.1)	0.44 (0.12-1.84, p=0.229)	0.37 (0.08-1.80, p=0.197)	-	-
	(50,75]	79 (76.0)	25 (24.0)	0.79 (0.24-3.08, p=0.712)	0.60 (0.15-2.65, p=0.469)	-	-
	(75,100]	9 (64.3)	5 (35.7)	1.39 (0.28-7.23, p=0.686)	0.61 (0.09-4.04, p=0.599)	-	-
Sex	Female	105 (83.3)	21 (16.7)	-	-	-	-
	Male	55 (69.6)	24 (30.4)	2.18 (1.12-4.30, p=0.023)	1.21 (0.54-2.68, p=0.633)	-	-
T-stage	T1	52 (92.9)	4 (7.1)	-	-	-	-
	T2	49 (92.5)	4 (7.5)	1.06 (0.24-4.71, p=0.936)	0.74 (0.15-3.50, p=0.697)	0.75 (0.16-3.45, p=0.700)	0.83 (0.18-3.73, p=0.807)
	T3	36 (70.6)	15 (29.4)	5.42 (1.80-20.22, p=0.005)	2.91 (0.84-11.82, p=0.106)	2.96 (0.86-11.96, p=0.098)	3.83 (1.00-14.70, p=0.051)
	T4	23 (51.1)	22 (48.9)	12.43 (4.21-46.26, p<0.001)	5.38 (1.43-23.52, p=0.016)	5.33 (1.48-22.56, p=0.014)	7.03 (1.71-28.86, p=0.007)

TABLE 9.18: Model metrics: multilevel (mixed effects) logistic regression.

Number in dataframe = 205, Number in model = 205, Missing = 0, AIC = 190, C-statistic = 0.802, H&L = Chi-sq(8) 13.87 (p=0.085)
Number in dataframe = 205, Number in model = 205, Missing = 0, AIC = 184.4, C-statistic = 0.791, H&L = Chi-sq(8) 0.43 (p=1.000)
Number in model = 205, Number of groups = 4, AIC = 173.2, C-statistic = 0.866

As can be seen, incorporating the (made-up) hospital identifier has altered our coefficients. It has also improved the model discrimination with a c-statistic of 0.830 from 0.802. Note that the AIC should not be used to compare mixed effects models estimated in this way with `glm()` models (the former uses a restricted maximum likelihood [REML] approach by default, while `glm()` uses maximum likelihood).

Random slope models are an extension of the random intercept model. Here the gradient of the response to a particular variable is allowed to vary by hospital. For example, this can be included using `random_effect = "(thickness | hospital_id)"` where the gradient of the continuous variable tumour thickness was allow to vary by hospital.

As models get more complex, care has to be taken to ensure the underlying data is understood and assumptions are checked.

Mixed effects modelling is a book in itself and the purpose here is to introduce the concept and provide some approaches for its incorporation. Clearly much is written elsewhere for those who are enthusiastic to learn more.

9.10   Exercises

9.10.1   Exercise

Investigate the association between sex and 5-year mortality for patients who have undergone surgery for melanoma.

First recode the variables as shown in the text, then plot the counts and proportions for 5-year disease-specific mortality in women and men. Is there an association between sex and mortality?

9.10.2 Exercise

Make a table showing the relationship between sex and the variables age, T-stage and ulceration. Hint: `summary_factorlist()`. Express age in terms of median and interquartile range. Include a statistical comparison.

What associations do you see?

9.10.3 Exercise

Run a logistic regression model for 5-year disease-specific mortality including sex, age, T-stage and ulceration.

What is the c-statistic for this model?

Is there a relationship between sex and mortality, after adjustment for the other explanatory variables?

9.10.4 Exercise

Make an odds ratio plot for this model.

9.11 Solutions

Solution to Exercise 9.10.1:

```
## Recode
melanoma <- melanoma %>%
  mutate(sex.factor = factor(sex) %>%
           fct_recode("Female" = "0",
                      "Male"   = "1") %>%
           ff_label("Sex"),

         ulcer.factor = factor(ulcer) %>%
           fct_recode("Present" = "1",
                      "Absent"  = "0") %>%
           ff_label("Ulcerated tumour"),

         age  = ff_label(age,  "Age (years)"),
```

```
        year = ff_label(year, "Year"),

        status.factor = factor(status) %>%
          fct_recode("Died melanoma"  = "1",
                     "Alive" = "2",
                     "Died - other" = "3") %>%
            fct_relevel("Alive") %>%
            ff_label("Status"),

        t_stage.factor =
          thickness %>%
          cut(breaks = c(0, 1.0, 2.0, 4.0,
                         max(thickness, na.rm=TRUE)),
              include.lowest = TRUE)
  )

# Plot
p1 <- melanoma %>%
  ggplot(aes(x = sex.factor, fill = mort_5yr)) +
  geom_bar() +
  theme(legend.position = "none")

p2 <- melanoma %>%
  ggplot(aes(x = sex.factor, fill = mort_5yr)) +
  geom_bar(position = "fill") +
  ylab("proportion")

p1 + p2
```

Solution to Exercise 9.10.2:

```
## Recode T-stage first
melanoma <- melanoma %>%
  mutate(
    t_stage.factor =
      fct_recode(t_stage.factor,
                 T1 = "[0,1]",
                 T2 = "(1,2]",
                 T3 = "(2,4]",
                 T4 = "(4,17.4]") %>%
        ff_label("T-stage")
  )

dependent = "sex.factor"
explanatory = c("age", "t_stage.factor", "ulcer.factor")
melanoma %>%
  summary_factorlist(dependent, explanatory, p = TRUE, na_include = TRUE,
                     cont = "median")

# Men have more T4 tumours and they are more likely to be ulcerated.
```

Solution to Exercise 9.10.3:

```
dependent = "mort_5yr"
explanatory = c("sex.factor", "age", "t_stage.factor", "ulcer.factor")
melanoma %>%
  finalfit(dependent, explanatory, metrics = TRUE)

# c-statistic = 0.798
# In multivariable model, male vs female OR 1.26 (0.57-2.76, p=0.558).
# No relationship after accounting for T-stage and tumour ulceration.
# Sex is confounded by these two variables.
```

Solution to Exercise 9.10.4:

```
dependent = "mort_5yr"
explanatory = c("sex.factor", "age", "t_stage.factor", "ulcer.factor")
melanoma %>%
  or_plot(dependent, explanatory)
```

10

Time-to-event data and survival

The reports of my death have been greatly exaggerated.
Mark Twain

In healthcare, we deal with a lot of binary outcomes. Death yes/no or disease recurrence yes/no for instance. These outcomes are often easily analysed using binary logistic regression as described in the previous chapter.

When the time taken for the outcome to occur is important, we need a different approach. For instance, in patients with cancer, the time taken until recurrence of the cancer is often just as important as the fact it has recurred.

10.1 The Question

We will again use the classic "Survival from Malignant Melanoma" dataset included in the **boot** package which we have used previously. The data consist of measurements made on patients with malignant melanoma. Each patient had their tumour removed by surgery at the Department of Plastic Surgery, University Hospital of Odense, Denmark, during the period 1962 to 1977.

We are interested in the association between tumour ulceration and survival after surgery.

10.2   Get and check the data

```
library(tidyverse)
library(finalfit)
melanoma <- boot::melanoma #F1 here for help page with data dictionary
```

```
glimpse(melanoma)
missing_glimpse(melanoma)
ff_glimpse(melanoma)
```

As was seen before, all variables are coded as numeric and some need recoding to factors. This is done below for those we are interested in.

10.3   Death status

`status` is the patient's status at the end of the study.

- 1 indicates that they had died from melanoma;
- 2 indicates that they were still alive and;
- 3 indicates that they had died from causes unrelated to their melanoma.

There are three options for coding this.

- Overall survival: considering all-cause mortality, comparing 2 (alive) with 1 (died melanoma)/3 (died other);
- Cause-specific survival: considering disease-specific mortality comparing 2 (alive)/3 (died other) with 1 (died melanoma);
- Competing risks: comparing 2 (alive) with 1 (died melanoma) accounting for 3 (died other); see more below.

10.4   Time and censoring

`time` is the number of days from surgery until either the occurrence of the event (death) or the last time the patient was known to be alive. For instance, if a patient had surgery and was seen to be well in a clinic 30 days later, but there had been no contact since, then the patient's status would be considered alive at 30 days. This patient is censored from the analysis at day 30, an important feature of time-to-event analyses.

10.5 Recode the data

```
library(dplyr)
library(forcats)
melanoma <- melanoma %>%
  mutate(
    # Overall survival
    status_os = if_else(status == 2, 0, # "still alive"
                        1), # "died of melanoma" or "died of other causes"

    # Diease-specific survival
    status_dss = if_else(status == 2, 0, # "still alive"
                         if_else(status == 1, 1, # "died of melanoma"
                                 0)), # "died of other causes is censored"

    # Competing risks regression
    status_crr = if_else(status == 2, 0, # "still alive"
                         if_else(status == 1, 1, # "died of melanoma"
                                 2)), # "died of other causes"

    # Label and recode other variables
    age = ff_label(age, "Age (years)"), # ff_label table friendly  labels
    thickness = ff_label(thickness, "Tumour thickness (mm)"),
    sex = factor(sex) %>%
      fct_recode("Male" = "1",
                 "Female" = "0") %>%
      ff_label("Sex"),
    ulcer = factor(ulcer) %>%
      fct_recode("No" = "0",
                 "Yes" = "1") %>%
      ff_label("Ulcerated tumour")
  )
```

10.6 Kaplan Meier survival estimator

We will use the excellent **survival** package to produce the Kaplan Meier (KM) survival estimator (Terry M. Therneau and Patricia M. Grambsch (2000), Therneau (2020)). This is a non-parametric statistic used to estimate the survival function from time-to-event data.

```r
library(survival)

survival_object <- melanoma %$%
    Surv(time, status_os)

# Explore:
head(survival_object) # + marks censoring, in this case "Alive"
```

```
## [1]  10   30   35+  99  185  204
```

```r
# Expressing time in years
survival_object <- melanoma %$%
    Surv(time/365, status_os)
```

10.6.1   KM analysis for whole cohort

10.6.2   Model

The survival object is the first step to performing univariable and multivariable survival analyses.

If you want to plot survival stratified by a single grouping variable, you can substitute "survival_object ~ 1" by "survival_object ~ factor"

```r
# Overall survival in whole cohort
my_survfit <- survfit(survival_object ~ 1, data = melanoma)
my_survfit # 205 patients, 71 events
```

```
## Call: survfit(formula = survival_object ~ 1, data = melanoma)
##
##        n   events  median 0.95LCL 0.95UCL
## 205.00   71.00      NA    9.15      NA
```

10.6.3   Life table

A life table is the tabular form of a KM plot, which you may be familiar with. It shows survival as a proportion, together with confidence limits. The whole table is shown with, summary(my_survfit).

```r
summary(my_survfit, times = c(0, 1, 2, 3, 4, 5))
```

```
## Call: survfit(formula = survival_object ~ 1, data = melanoma)
##
##  time n.risk n.event survival std.err lower 95% CI upper 95% CI
##     0    205       0    1.000  0.0000        1.000        1.000
##     1    193      11    0.946  0.0158        0.916        0.978
##     2    183      10    0.897  0.0213        0.856        0.940
```

```
##    3    167    16    0.819  0.0270       0.767         0.873
##    4    160     7    0.784  0.0288       0.730         0.843
##    5    122    10    0.732  0.0313       0.673         0.796


# 5 year overall survival is 73%
```

10.7 Kaplan Meier plot

We can plot survival curves using the **finalfit** wrapper for the package **survminer**. There are numerous options available on the help page. You should always include a number-at-risk table under these plots as it is essential for interpretation.

As can be seen, the probability of dying is much greater if the tumour was ulcerated, compared to those that were not ulcerated.

```
dependent_os <- "Surv(time/365, status_os)"
explanatory  <- c("ulcer")

melanoma %>%
    surv_plot(dependent_os, explanatory, pval = TRUE)


## Warning: Vectorized input to `element_text()` is not officially supported.
## Results may be unexpected or may change in future versions of ggplot2.
```

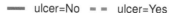

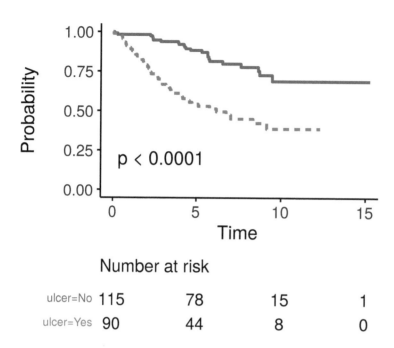

10.8   Cox proportional hazards regression

The Cox proportional hazards model is a regression model similar to those we have already dealt with. It is commonly used to investigate the association between the time to an event (such as death) and a set of explanatory variables.

Cox proportional hazards regression can be performed using `survival::coxph()` or the all-in-one `finalfit()` function. The latter produces a table containing counts (proportions) for factors, mean (SD) for continuous variables and a univariable and multivariable CPH regression.

10.8.1   `coxph()`

CPH using the `coxph()` function produces a similar output to `lm()` and `glm()`, so it should be familiar to you now. It can be passed to `summary()` as below, and also to `broom::tidy()` if you want to get the results into a tibble.

```
library(survival)
coxph(Surv(time, status_os) ~ age + sex + thickness + ulcer, data = melanoma) %>%
  summary()
```

```
## Call:
## coxph(formula = Surv(time, status_os) ~ age + sex + thickness +
##     ulcer, data = melanoma)
##
##   n= 205, number of events= 71
##
##                coef exp(coef) se(coef)     z Pr(>|z|)
## age        0.021831  1.022071 0.007752 2.816 0.004857 **
## sexMale    0.413460  1.512040 0.240132 1.722 0.085105 .
## thickness  0.099467  1.104582 0.034455 2.887 0.003891 **
## ulcerYes   0.952083  2.591100 0.267966 3.553 0.000381 ***
## ---
## Signif. codes:  0 '***' 0.001 '**' 0.01 '*' 0.05 '.' 0.1 ' ' 1
##
##            exp(coef) exp(-coef) lower .95 upper .95
## age            1.022     0.9784    1.0067     1.038
## sexMale        1.512     0.6614    0.9444     2.421
## thickness      1.105     0.9053    1.0325     1.182
## ulcerYes       2.591     0.3859    1.5325     4.381
##
## Concordance= 0.739  (se = 0.03 )
## Likelihood ratio test= 47.89  on 4 df,   p=1e-09
## Wald test            = 46.72  on 4 df,   p=2e-09
## Score (logrank) test = 52.77  on 4 df,   p=1e-10
```

The output shows the number of patients and the number of events. The coefficient can be exponentiated and interpreted as a **hazard ratio**, exp(coef). Helpfully, 95% confidence intervals are also provided.

A hazard is the term given to the rate at which events happen. The probability that an event will happen over a period of time is the hazard multiplied by the time interval. An assumption of CPH is that hazards are constant over time (see below).

For a given predictor then, the hazard in one group (say males) would be expected to be a constant proportion of the hazard in another group (say females). The ratio of these hazards is, unsurprisingly, the hazard ratio.

The hazard ratio differs from the relative risk and odds ratio. The hazard ratio represents the difference in the risk of an event at any given time, whereas the relative risk or odds ratio usually represents the cumulative risk over a period of time.

10.8.2 finalfit()

Alternatively, a CPH regression can be run with **finalfit** functions. This is convenient for model fitting, exploration and the export of results.

```
dependent_os  <- "Surv(time, status_os)"
dependent_dss <- "Surv(time, status_dss)"
dependent_crr <- "Surv(time, status_crr)"
```

```
explanatory    <- c("age", "sex", "thickness", "ulcer")

melanoma %>%
    finalfit(dependent_os, explanatory)
```

The labelling of the final table can be adjusted as desired.

```
melanoma %>%
    finalfit(dependent_os, explanatory, add_dependent_label = FALSE) %>%
    rename("Overall survival" = label) %>%
    rename(" " = levels) %>%
    rename("  " = all)
```

TABLE 10.1: Univariable and multivariable Cox Proportional Hazards: Overall survival following surgery for melanoma by patient and tumour variables (tidied).

Overall survival			HR (univariable)	HR (multivariable)
Age (years)	Mean (SD)	52.5 (16.7)	1.03 (1.01-1.05, p<0.001)	1.02 (1.01-1.04, p=0.005)
Sex	Female	126 (100.0)	-	-
	Male	79 (100.0)	1.93 (1.21-3.07, p=0.006)	1.51 (0.94-2.42, p=0.085)
Tumour thickness (mm)	Mean (SD)	2.9 (3.0)	1.16 (1.10-1.23, p<0.001)	1.10 (1.03-1.18, p=0.004)
Ulcerated tumour	No	115 (100.0)	-	-
	Yes	90 (100.0)	3.52 (2.14-5.80, p<0.001)	2.59 (1.53-4.38, p<0.001)

10.8.3 Reduced model

If you are using a backwards selection approach or similar, a reduced model can be directly specified and compared. The full model can be kept or dropped.

```
explanatory_multi <- c("age", "thickness", "ulcer")
melanoma %>%
    finalfit(dependent_os, explanatory,
             explanatory_multi, keep_models = TRUE)
```

TABLE 10.2: Cox Proportional Hazards: Overall survival following surgery for melanoma with reduced model.

Dependent: Surv(time, status_os)		all	HR (univariable)	HR (multivariable)	HR (multivariable reduced)
Age (years)	Mean (SD)	52.5 (16.7)	1.03 (1.01-1.05, p<0.001)	1.02 (1.01-1.04, p=0.005)	1.02 (1.01-1.04, p=0.003)
Sex	Female	126 (100.0)	-	-	
	Male	79 (100.0)	1.93 (1.21-3.07, p=0.006)	1.51 (0.94-2.42, p=0.085)	-
Tumour thickness (mm)	Mean (SD)	2.9 (3.0)	1.16 (1.10-1.23, p<0.001)	1.10 (1.03-1.18, p=0.004)	1.10 (1.03-1.18, p=0.003)
Ulcerated tumour	No	115 (100.0)	-	-	
	Yes	90 (100.0)	3.52 (2.14-5.80, p<0.001)	2.59 (1.53-4.38, p<0.001)	2.72 (1.61-4.57, p<0.001)

10.8.4 Testing for proportional hazards

An assumption of CPH regression is that the hazard (think risk) associated with a particular variable does not change over time. For example, is the magnitude of the increase in risk of death associated with tumour ulceration the same in the early post-operative period as it is in later years?

The `cox.zph()` function from the **survival** package allows us to test this assumption for each variable. The plot of scaled Schoenfeld residuals should be a horizontal line. The included hypothesis test identifies whether the gradient differs from zero for each variable. No variable significantly differs from zero at the 5% significance level.

```
explanatory <- c("age", "sex", "thickness", "ulcer", "year")
melanoma %>%
    coxphmulti(dependent_os, explanatory) %>%
    cox.zph() %>%
    {zph_result <<- .} %>%
    plot(var=5)
```

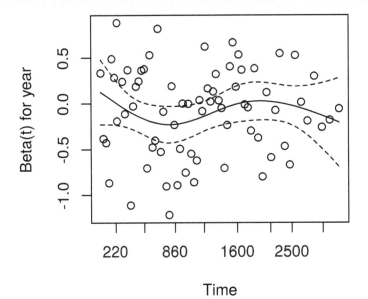

```
zph_result
```

```
##             chisq df     p
## age         2.067  1 0.151
## sex         0.505  1 0.477
## thickness   2.837  1 0.092
## ulcer       4.325  1 0.038
## year        0.451  1 0.502
## GLOBAL      7.891  5 0.162
```

10.8.5   Stratified models

One approach to dealing with a violation of the proportional hazards assumption is to stratify by that variable. Including a `strata()` term will result in a separate baseline hazard function being fit for each level in the stratification variable. It will be no longer possible to make direct inference on the effect associated with that variable.

This can be incorporated directly into the explanatory variable list.

```
explanatory <- c("age", "sex", "ulcer", "thickness",
                 "strata(year)")
melanoma %>%
    finalfit(dependent_os, explanatory)
```

TABLE 10.3: Cox Proportional Hazards: Overall survival following surgery for melanoma stratified by year of surgery.

Dependent: Surv(time, status_os)		all	HR (univariable)	HR (multivariable)
Age (years)	Mean (SD)	52.5 (16.7)	1.03 (1.01-1.05, p<0.001)	1.03 (1.01-1.05, p=0.002)
Sex	Female	126 (100.0)	-	-
	Male	79 (100.0)	1.93 (1.21-3.07, p=0.006)	1.75 (1.06-2.87, p=0.027)
Ulcerated tumour	No	115 (100.0)	-	-
	Yes	90 (100.0)	3.52 (2.14-5.80, p<0.001)	2.61 (1.47-4.63, p=0.001)
Tumour thickness (mm)	Mean (SD)	2.9 (3.0)	1.16 (1.10-1.23, p<0.001)	1.08 (1.01-1.16, p=0.027)
strata(year)			-	-

10.8.6   Correlated groups of observations

As a general rule, you should always try to account for any higher structure in your data within the model. For instance, patients may be clustered within particular hospitals.

There are two broad approaches to dealing with correlated groups of observations.

Adding a `cluster()` term is similar to a generalised estimating equations (GEE) approach (something we're not covering in this book). Here, a standard CPH model is fitted but the standard errors of the estimated hazard ratios are adjusted to account for correlations.

A `frailty()` term implies a mixed effects model, where specific random effects term(s) are directly incorporated into the model.

Both approaches achieve the same goal in different ways. Volumes have been written on GEE vs mixed effects models and we won't rehearse them in this introductory book. We favour the latter approach because of its flexibility and our preference for mixed effects modelling in generalised linear modelling. Note `cluster()` and `frailty()` terms cannot be combined in the same model.

```
# Simulate random hospital identifier
melanoma <- melanoma %>%
    mutate(hospital_id = c(rep(1:10, 20), rep(11, 5)))

# Cluster model
explanatory <- c("age", "sex", "thickness", "ulcer",
                "cluster(hospital_id)")
melanoma %>%
    finalfit(dependent_os, explanatory)
```

TABLE 10.4: Cox Proportional Hazards: Overall survival following surgery for melanoma with robust standard errors (cluster model).

Dependent: Surv(time, status_os)		all	HR (univariable)	HR (multivariable)
Age (years)	Mean (SD)	52.5 (16.7)	1.03 (1.01-1.05, p<0.001)	1.02 (1.00-1.04, p=0.016)
Sex	Female	126 (100.0)	-	-
	Male	79 (100.0)	1.93 (1.21-3.07, p=0.006)	1.51 (1.10-2.08, p=0.011)
Tumour thickness (mm)	Mean (SD)	2.9 (3.0)	1.16 (1.10-1.23, p<0.001)	1.10 (1.04-1.17, p<0.001)
Ulcerated tumour	No	115 (100.0)	-	-
	Yes	90 (100.0)	3.52 (2.14-5.80, p<0.001)	2.59 (1.61-4.16, p<0.001)
cluster(hospital_id)			-	-

```
# Frailty model
explanatory <- c("age", "sex", "thickness", "ulcer",
                "frailty(hospital_id)")
melanoma %>%
    finalfit(dependent_os, explanatory)
```

TABLE 10.5: Cox Proportional Hazards: Overall survival following surgery for melanoma (frailty model).

Dependent: Surv(time, status_os)		all	HR (univariable)	HR (multivariable)
Age (years)	Mean (SD)	52.5 (16.7)	1.03 (1.01-1.05, p<0.001)	1.02 (1.01-1.04, p=0.005)
Sex	Female	126 (100.0)	-	-
	Male	79 (100.0)	1.93 (1.21-3.07, p=0.006)	1.51 (0.94-2.42, p=0.085)
Tumour thickness (mm)	Mean (SD)	2.9 (3.0)	1.16 (1.10-1.23, p<0.001)	1.10 (1.03-1.18, p=0.004)
Ulcerated tumour	No	115 (100.0)	-	-
	Yes	90 (100.0)	3.52 (2.14-5.80, p<0.001)	2.59 (1.53-4.38, p<0.001)
frailty(hospital_id)			-	-

The `frailty()` method here is being superseded by the **coxme** package, and we look forward to incorporating this in the future.

10.8.7 Hazard ratio plot

A plot of any of the above models can be produced using the `hr_plot()` function.

```
melanoma %>%
    hr_plot(dependent_os, explanatory)
```

10.9   Competing risks regression

Competing-risks regression is an alternative to CPH regression. It can be useful if the outcome of interest may not be able to occur simply because something else (like death) has happened first. For instance, in our example it is obviously not possible for a patient to die from melanoma if they have died from another disease first. By simply looking at cause-specific mortality (deaths from melanoma) and considering other deaths as censored, bias may result in estimates of the influence of predictors.

The approach by Fine and Gray is one option for dealing with this. It is implemented in the package **cmprsk**. The `crr()` syntax differs from `survival::coxph()` but `finalfit` brings these together.

It uses the `finalfit::ff_merge()` function, which can join any number of models together.

```
explanatory   <- c("age", "sex", "thickness", "ulcer")
dependent_dss <- "Surv(time, status_dss)"
dependent_crr <- "Surv(time, status_crr)"

melanoma %>%
    # Summary table
  summary_factorlist(dependent_dss, explanatory,
                     column = TRUE, fit_id = TRUE) %>%
    # CPH univariable
    ff_merge(
    melanoma %>%
    coxphmulti(dependent_dss, explanatory) %>%
    fit2df(estimate_suffix = " (DSS CPH univariable)")
  ) %>%
    # CPH multivariable
  ff_merge(
    melanoma %>%
    coxphmulti(dependent_dss, explanatory) %>%
    fit2df(estimate_suffix = " (DSS CPH multivariable)")
  ) %>%
    # Fine and Gray competing risks regression
  ff_merge(
    melanoma %>%
    crrmulti(dependent_crr, explanatory) %>%
    fit2df(estimate_suffix = " (competing risks multivariable)")
  ) %>%
```

```
select(-fit_id, -index) %>%
dependent_label(melanoma, "Survival")
```

```
## Dependent variable is a survival object
```

TABLE 10.6: Cox Proportional Hazards and competing risks regression combined.

Dependent: Survival		all	HR (DSS CPH univariable)	HR (DSS CPH multivariable)	HR (competing risks multivariable)
Age (years)	Mean (SD)	52.5 (16.7)	1.01 (1.00-1.03, p=0.141)	1.01 (1.00-1.03, p=0.141)	1.01 (0.99-1.02, p=0.520)
Sex	Female	126 (61.5)	-	-	-
	Male	79 (38.5)	1.54 (0.91-2.60, p=0.106)	1.54 (0.91-2.60, p=0.106)	1.50 (0.87-2.57, p=0.140)
Tumour thickness (mm)	Mean (SD)	2.9 (3.0)	1.12 (1.04-1.20, p=0.004)	1.12 (1.04-1.20, p=0.004)	1.09 (1.01-1.18, p=0.019)
Ulcerated tumour	No	115 (56.1)	-	-	-
	Yes	90 (43.9)	3.20 (1.75-5.88, p<0.001)	3.20 (1.75-5.88, p<0.001)	3.09 (1.71-5.60, p<0.001)

10.10 Summary

So here we have presented the various aspects of time-to-event analysis which are commonly used when looking at survival. There are many other applications, some of which may not be obvious: for instance we use CPH for modelling length of stay in hospital.

Stratification can be used to deal with non-proportional hazards in a particular variable.

Hierarchical structure in your data can be accommodated with cluster or frailty (random effects) terms.

Competing risks regression may be useful if your outcome is in competition with another, such as all-cause death, but is currently limited in its ability to accommodate hierarchical structures.

10.11 Dates in R

10.11.1 Converting dates to survival time

In the melanoma example dataset, we already had the time in a convenient format for survival analysis - survival time in days since the operation. This section shows how to convert dates into "days from event". First we will generate a dummy operation date and censoring date based on the melanoma data.

```
library(lubridate)
first_date <- ymd("1966-01-01")          # create made-up dates for operations
last_date  <- first_date +
  days(nrow(melanoma)-1)                  # every day from 1-Jan 1966
operation_date <-
  seq(from = first_date,
      to = last_date, by = "1 day")       # create dates

melanoma$operation_date <- operation_date # add sequence to melanoma dataset
```

Now we will create a 'censoring' date by adding `time` from the melanoma dataset to our made up operation date.

Remember the censoring date is either when an event occurred (e.g., death) or the last known alive status of the patient.

```
melanoma <- melanoma %>%
  mutate(censoring_date = operation_date + days(time))

# (Same as doing:):
melanoma$censoring_date <- melanoma$operation_date + days(melanoma$time)
```

Now consider if we only had the `operation` date and `censoring` date. We want to create the `time` variable.

```
melanoma <- melanoma %>%
  mutate(time_days = censoring_date - operation_date)
```

The `Surv()` function expects a number (`numeric` variable), rather than a `date` object, so we'll convert it:

```
# This doesn't work
# Surv(melanoma$time_days, melanoma$status==1)
melanoma <- melanoma %>%
  mutate(time_days_numeric = as.numeric(time_days))

# This works as exepcted.
Surv(melanoma$time_days_numeric, melanoma$status.factor == "Died")
```

10.12   Exercises

10.12.1   Exercise

Using the above scripts, perform a univariable Kaplan Meier analysis to determine if `ulcer` influences overall survival. Hint: `survival_object ~ ulcer`.

Try modifying the plot produced (see Help for ggsurvplot). For example:

- Add in a median survival line: `surv.median.line="hv"`
- Alter the plot legend: `legend.title = "Ulcer Present"`, `legend.labs = c("No", "Yes")`
- Change the y-axis to a percentage: `ylab = "Probability of survival (%)"`, `surv.scale = "percent"`
- Display follow-up up to 10 years, and change the scale to 1 year: `xlim = c(0,10)`, `break.time.by = 1`

10.12.2   Exercise

Create a new CPH model, but now include the variable `thickness` as a variable.

- How would you interpret the output?
- Is it an independent predictor of overall survival in this model?
- Are CPH assumptions maintained?

10.13   Solutions

Solution to Exercise 10.12.1:

```
## Call: survfit(formula = survival_object ~ ulcer, data = melanoma)
##
##                   ulcer=No
##  time n.risk n.event survival std.err lower 95% CI upper 95% CI
##    0    115       0    1.000   0.0000       1.000        1.000
##    1    112       2    0.983   0.0122       0.959        1.000
##    2    112       0    0.983   0.0122       0.959        1.000
##    3    107       5    0.939   0.0225       0.896        0.984
##    4    105       2    0.921   0.0252       0.873        0.972
##    5     78       4    0.883   0.0306       0.825        0.945
##
##                   ulcer=Yes
##  time n.risk n.event survival std.err lower 95% CI upper 95% CI
##    0     90       0    1.000   0.0000       1.000        1.000
##    1     81       9    0.900   0.0316       0.840        0.964
##    2     71      10    0.789   0.0430       0.709        0.878
##    3     60      11    0.667   0.0497       0.576        0.772
##    4     55       5    0.611   0.0514       0.518        0.721
```

```
##     5    44      6   0.543  0.0526       0.449        0.657
## Warning: Vectorized input to `element_text()` is not officially supported.
## Results may be unexpected or may change in future versions of ggplot2.
```

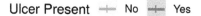

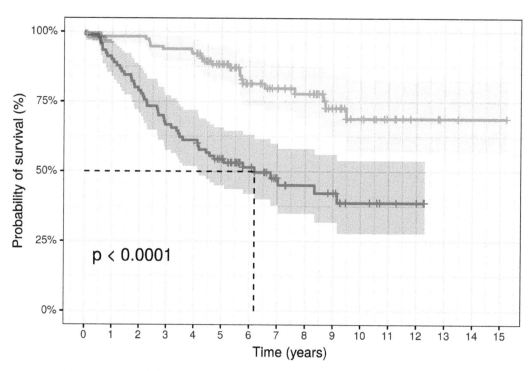

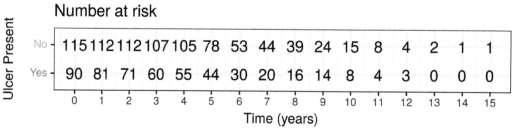

Solution to Exercise 10.12.2:

```
# Fit model
my_hazard = coxph(survival_object ~ sex + ulcer + age + thickness, data=melanoma)
summary(my_hazard)

# Melanoma thickness has a HR 1.11 (1.03 to 1.18).
# This is interpretted as a 11% increase in the
# risk of death at any time for each 1 mm increase in thickness.

# Check assumptions
ph = cox.zph(my_hazard)
ph
# GLOBAL shows no overall violation of assumptions.
```

```
# Plot Schoenfield residuals to evaluate PH
plot(ph, var=4)
```

Part III

Workflow

Throughout this book we have tried to provide the most efficient approaches to data analysis using R. In this section, we will provide workflows, or ways-of-working, which maximise efficiency, incorporate reporting of results within analyses, make exporting of tables and plots easy, and keep data safe, secured and backed up.

We also include a section on dealing with missing data in R. Something that we both feel strongly about and which is often poorly described and dealt with in academic publishing.

11

The problem of missing data

In heaven, all the interesting people are missing.
Friedrich Nietzsche

11.1 Identification of missing data

As journal editors, we often receive studies in which the investigators fail to describe, analyse, or even acknowledge missing data. This is frustrating, as it is often of the utmost importance. Conclusions may (and do) change when missing data are accounted for. Some folk seem to not even appreciate that in a conventional regression, only rows with complete data are included. By reading this, you will not be one of them!

These are the five steps to ensuring missing data are correctly identified and appropriately dealt with:

1. Ensure your data are coded correctly.
2. Identify missing values within each variable.
3. Look for patterns of missingness.
4. Check for associations between missing and observed data.
5. Decide how to handle missing data.

We will work through a number of functions that will help with each of these. But first, here are some terms that are easy to mix up. These are important as they describe the mechanism of missingness and this determines how you can handle the missing data.

For each of the following examples we will imagine that we are collecting data on the relationship between gender, smoking and the outcome of cancer treatment. The ground truth in this imagined scenario is that both gender and smoking influence the outcome from cancer treatment.

11.1.1 Missing completely at random (MCAR)

As it says, values are randomly missing from your dataset. Missing data values do not relate to any other data in the dataset and there is no pattern to the actual values of the missing data themselves.

In our example, smoking status is missing from a random subset of male and female patients.

This may have the effect of making our population smaller, but the complete case population has the same characteristics as the missing data population. This is easy to handle, but unfortunately, data are almost never missing completely at random.

11.1.2 Missing at random (MAR)

This is confusing and would be better named *missing conditionally at random*. Here, missingness in a particular variable has an association with one or more other variables in the dataset. However, the *actual values of the missing data are random*.

In our example, smoking status is missing for some female patients but not for male patients.

But data is missing from the same number of female smokers as female non-smokers. So the complete case female patients has the same characteristics as the missing data female patients.

11.1.3 Missing not at random (MNAR)

The pattern of missingness is related to other variables in the dataset, but in addition, the *actual values of the missing data are not random*.

In our example, smoking status is missing in female patients who are more likely to smoke, but not for male patients.

Thus, the complete case female patients have different characteristics to the missing data female patients. For instance, the missing data female patients may be more likely to die after cancer treatment. Looking at our available population, we therefore under estimate the likelihood of a female dying from cancer treatment.

Missing not at random data are important, can alter your conclusions, and are the most difficult to diagnose and handle. They can only be detected by collecting and examining some of the missing data. This is often difficult or impossible to do.

How you deal with missing data is dependent on the type of missingness. Once you know the type, you can start addressing it. More on this below.

11.2 Ensure your data are coded correctly: `ff_glimpse()`

While it sounds obvious, this step is often ignored in the rush to get results. The first step in any analysis is robust data cleaning and coding. Lots of packages have a glimpse-type function and our own **finalfit** is no different. This function has three specific goals:

1. Ensure all variables are of the type you expect them to be. That is the commonest reason to get an error with a **finalfit** function. Numbers should be numeric, categorical variables should be characters or factors, and dates should be dates (for a reminder on these, see Section 2.2.

2. Ensure you know which variables have missing data. This presumes missing values are correctly assigned NA.

3. Ensure factor levels and variable labels are assigned correctly.

11.2.1 The Question

Using the `colon_s` colon cancer dataset, we are interested in exploring the association between a cancer obstructing the bowel and 5-year survival, accounting for other patient and disease characteristics.

For demonstration purposes, we will make up MCAR and MAR smoking variables (`smoking_mcar` and `smoking_mar`). Do not worry about understanding the long cascading mutate and `sample()` functions below, this is merely for creating the example variables. You would not be 'creating' your data, we hope.

```
# Create some extra missing data
library(finalfit)
library(dplyr)
set.seed(1)
colon_s <- colon_s %>%
  mutate(
    ## Smoking missing completely at random
    smoking_mcar = sample(c("Smoker", "Non-smoker", NA),
                          n(), replace=TRUE,
                          prob = c(0.2, 0.7, 0.1)) %>%
      factor() %>%
      ff_label("Smoking (MCAR)"),
```

```
## Smoking missing conditional on patient sex
smoking_mar = ifelse(sex.factor == "Female",
                  sample(c("Smoker", "Non-smoker", NA),
                      sum(sex.factor == "Female"),
                      replace = TRUE,
                      prob = c(0.1, 0.5, 0.4)),

                  sample(c("Smoker", "Non-smoker", NA),
                      sum(sex.factor == "Male"),
                      replace=TRUE, prob = c(0.15, 0.75, 0.1))
) %>%
    factor() %>%
    ff_label("Smoking (MAR)")
)
```

We will then examine our variables of interest using `ff_glimpse()`:

```
explanatory <- c("age", "sex.factor",
              "nodes", "obstruct.factor",
              "smoking_mcar", "smoking_mar")
dependent <- "mort_5yr"

colon_s %>%
  ff_glimpse(dependent, explanatory)
```

```
## $Continuous
##             label var_type   n missing_n missing_percent mean   sd  min
## age   Age (years)    <dbl> 929         0             0.0 59.8 11.9 18.0
## nodes       nodes    <dbl> 911        18             1.9  3.7  3.6  0.0
##       quartile_25 median quartile_75  max
## age          53.0   61.0        69.0 85.0
## nodes         1.0    2.0         5.0 33.0
##
## $Categorical
##                        label var_type   n missing_n missing_percent
## mort_5yr     Mortality 5 year    <fct> 915        14             1.5
## sex.factor                Sex    <fct> 929         0             0.0
## obstruct.factor   Obstruction    <fct> 908        21             2.3
## smoking_mcar    Smoking (MCAR)    <fct> 828       101            10.9
## smoking_mar      Smoking (MAR)    <fct> 726       203            21.9
##                 levels_n                              levels  levels_count
## mort_5yr               2          "Alive", "Died", "(Missing)"  511, 404, 14
## sex.factor            2                      "Female", "Male"      445, 484
## obstruct.factor       2          "No", "Yes", "(Missing)"   732, 176, 21
## smoking_mcar          2 "Non-smoker", "Smoker", "(Missing)" 645, 183, 101
## smoking_mar           2 "Non-smoker", "Smoker", "(Missing)" 585, 141, 203
##                 levels_percent
## mort_5yr         55.0, 43.5,  1.5
## sex.factor               48, 52
## obstruct.factor 78.8, 18.9,  2.3
## smoking_mcar         69, 20, 11
## smoking_mar          63, 15, 22
```

You don't need to specify the variables, and if you don't, `ff_glimpse()` will summarise all variables:

```
colon_s %>%
  ff_glimpse()
```

Use this to check that the variables are all assigned and behaving as expected. The proportion of missing data can be seen, e.g., `smoking_mar` has 22% missing data.

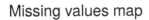

11.3 Identify missing values in each variable: `missing_plot()`

Visualising data is essential to help understand it, and missing data is no exception. `missing_plot()` function also from **finalfit** is useful for grasping the amount of missing data in each variable. Row number is on the x-axis and all included variables are on the y-axis.

```
colon_s %>%
  missing_plot(dependent, explanatory)
```

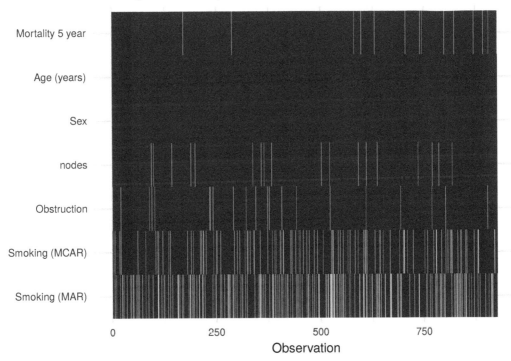

Further visualisations of missingness can be done using the naniar[1] package.

---
[1] http://naniar.njtierney.com

11.4 Look for patterns of missingness: `missing_pattern()`

Using **finalfit**, `missing_pattern()` wraps a function from the **mice** package, `md.pattern()`. This produces a table and a plot showing the pattern of missingness between variables.

```
explanatory <- c("age", "sex.factor",
                 "obstruct.factor",
                 "smoking_mcar", "smoking_mar")
dependent <- "mort_5yr"

colon_s %>%
  missing_pattern(dependent, explanatory)
```

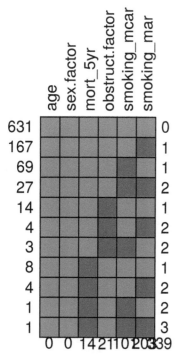

```
##      age sex.factor mort_5yr obstruct.factor smoking_mcar smoking_mar
## 631    1          1        1               1            1           1   0
## 167    1          1        1               1            1           0   1
## 69     1          1        1               1            0           1   1
## 27     1          1        1               1            0           0   2
## 14     1          1        1               0            1           1   1
## 4      1          1        1               0            1           0   2
## 3      1          1        1               0            0           1   2
## 8      1          1        0               1            1           1   1
## 4      1          1        0               1            1           0   2
## 1      1          1        0               1            0           1   2
## 1      1          1        0               1            0           0   3
##        0          0       14              21          101         203 339
```

This allows us to look for patterns of missingness between variables. There are 11 patterns in these data. The number and pattern of missingness help us to determine the likelihood of it being random rather than systematic.

11.5 Including missing data in demographics tables

"Table 1" in a healthcare study is often a demographics table of an "explanatory variable of interest" against other explanatory variables/confounders. Do not silently drop missing values in this table. It is easy to do this correctly with `summary_factorlist()`. This function provides a useful summary of a dependent variable against explanatory variables. Despite its name, continuous variables are handled nicely.

`na_include=TRUE` ensures missing data from the explanatory variables (but not dependent) are included. To include missing values from the dependent, add `na_include_dependent = TRUE`. Including a total column (`total_col = TRUE`) is also useful, as well as column totals (`add_col_totals = TRUE`).

If you are using a lot of continuous explanatory variables with missing values, then these can be seen easily using `add_row_totals = TRUE`.

Note that missing data is not included when p-values are generated. If you wish missing data to be passed to statistical tests, then include `na_to_p = TRUE`.

```
# Explanatory or confounding variables
explanatory <- c("age", "sex.factor",
                 "nodes",
                 "smoking_mcar", "smoking_mar")

# Explanatory variable of interest
dependent <- "obstruct.factor" # Bowel obstruction

table1 <- colon_s %>%
  summary_factorlist(dependent, explanatory,
                     na_include=TRUE, na_include_dependent = TRUE,
                     total_col = TRUE, add_col_totals = TRUE, p=TRUE)
```

11.6 Check for associations between missing and observed data

In deciding whether data is MCAR or MAR, one approach is to explore patterns of missingness between levels of included variables. This is particularly

TABLE 11.1: Simulated missing completely at random (MCAR) and missing at random (MAR) dataset.

label	levels	No	Yes	(Missing)	Total	p
Total N (%)		732 (78.8)	176 (18.9)	21 (2.3)	929	
Age (years)	Mean (SD)	60.2 (11.5)	57.3 (13.3)	63.9 (11.9)	59.8 (11.9)	0.004
Sex	Female	346 (47.3)	91 (51.7)	8 (38.1)	445 (47.9)	0.330
	Male	386 (52.7)	85 (48.3)	13 (61.9)	484 (52.1)	
nodes	Mean (SD)	3.7 (3.7)	3.5 (3.2)	3.3 (3.1)	3.7 (3.6)	0.435
Smoking (MCAR)	Non-smoker	500 (68.3)	130 (73.9)	15 (71.4)	645 (69.4)	0.080
	Smoker	154 (21.0)	26 (14.8)	3 (14.3)	183 (19.7)	
	(Missing)	78 (10.7)	20 (11.4)	3 (14.3)	101 (10.9)	
Smoking (MAR)	Non-smoker	456 (62.3)	115 (65.3)	14 (66.7)	585 (63.0)	0.822
	Smoker	112 (15.3)	26 (14.8)	3 (14.3)	141 (15.2)	
	(Missing)	164 (22.4)	35 (19.9)	4 (19.0)	203 (21.9)	

important (we would say absolutely required) for a primary outcome measure / dependent variable.

Take for example "death". When that outcome is missing it is often for a particular reason. For example, perhaps patients undergoing emergency surgery were less likely to have complete records compared with those undergoing planned surgery. And of course, death is more likely after emergency surgery.

`missing_pairs()` uses functions from the **GGally** package. It produces pairs plots to show relationships between missing values and observed values in all variables.

```
explanatory <- c("age", "sex.factor",
                 "nodes", "obstruct.factor",
                 "smoking_mcar", "smoking_mar")
dependent <- "mort_5yr"
colon_s %>%
  missing_pairs(dependent, explanatory)
```

For continuous variables (age and nodes), the distributions of observed and missing data can immediately be visually compared. For example, look at Row 1 Column 2. The age of patients who's mortality data is known is the blue box plot, and the age of patients with missing mortality data is the grey box plot.

For categorical data, the comparisons are presented as counts (remember `geom_bar()` from Chapter 4). To be able to compare proportions, we can add the `position = "fill"` argument:

```
colon_s %>%
  missing_pairs(dependent, explanatory, position = "fill")
```

Missing data matrix

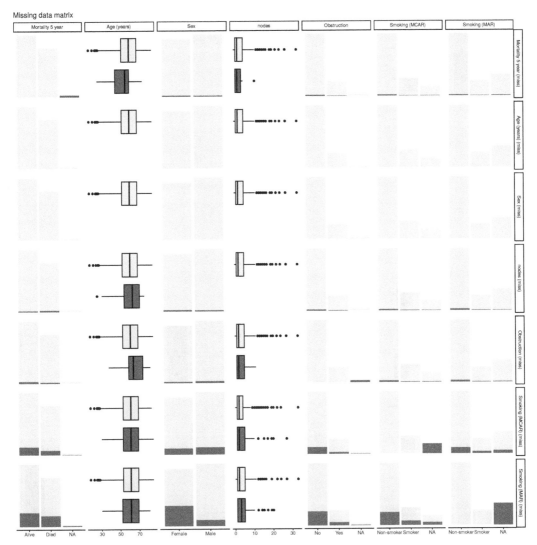

FIGURE 11.1: Missing data matrix with `missing_pairs()`.

Find the two sets of bar plots that show the proportion of missing smoking data for sex (bottom of Column 3). Missingness in Smoking (MCAR) does not relate to sex - females and males have the same proportion of missing data. Missingness in Smoking (MAR), however, does differ by sex as females have more missing data than men here. This is how we designed the example at the top of this chapter, so it all makes sense.

We can also confirm this by using `missing_compare()`:

```
explanatory <- c("age", "sex.factor",
                 "nodes", "obstruct.factor")
dependent <- "smoking_mcar"
```

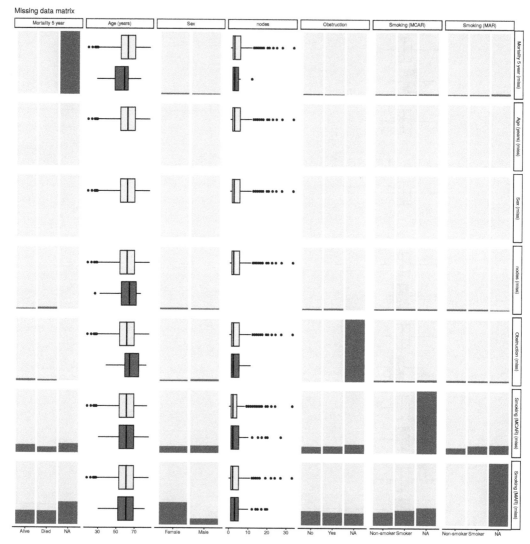

FIGURE 11.2: Missing data matrix with `missing_pairs(position = 'fill')` .

```
missing_mcar <- colon_s %>%
  missing_compare(dependent, explanatory)
```

TABLE 11.2: Missing data comparison: Smoking (MCAR).

Missing data analysis: Smoking (MCAR)		Not missing	Missing	p
Age (years)	Mean (SD)	59.7 (11.9)	59.9 (12.6)	0.882
Sex	Female	399 (89.7)	46 (10.3)	0.692
	Male	429 (88.6)	55 (11.4)	
nodes	Mean (SD)	3.6 (3.4)	4.0 (4.5)	0.302
Obstruction	No	654 (89.3)	78 (10.7)	0.891
	Yes	156 (88.6)	20 (11.4)	

```
dependent <- "smoking_mar"

missing_mar <- colon_s %>%
  missing_compare(dependent, explanatory)
```

TABLE 11.3: Missing data comparison: Smoking (MAR).

Missing data analysis: Smoking (MAR)		Not missing	Missing	p
Age (years)	Mean (SD)	59.9 (11.8)	59.4 (12.6)	0.632
Sex	Female	288 (64.7)	157 (35.3)	<0.001
	Male	438 (90.5)	46 (9.5)	
nodes	Mean (SD)	3.6 (3.5)	3.9 (3.9)	0.321
Obstruction	No	568 (77.6)	164 (22.4)	0.533
	Yes	141 (80.1)	35 (19.9)	

It takes dependent and explanatory variables, and in this context "dependent" refers to the variable being tested for missingness against the explanatory variables. [2] As expected, a relationship is seen between sex and smoking (MAR) but not smoking (MCAR).

11.6.1 For those who like an omnibus test

If you work predominately with continuous rather than categorical data, you may find these tests from the MissMech package useful. It provides two tests which can be used to determine whether data are MCAR; the package and its output are well documented.

```
library(MissMech)
explanatory <- c("age", "nodes")
dependent <- "mort_5yr"

colon_s %>%
  select(all_of(explanatory)) %>%
  MissMech::TestMCARNormality()

## Call:
## MissMech::TestMCARNormality(data = .)
##
## Number of Patterns:  2
##
## Total number of cases used in the analysis:  929
##
##   Pattern(s) used:
##           age    nodes    Number of cases
```

---

[2]By default, missing_compare() uses an F-test test for continuous variables and chi-squared for categorical variables; you can change these the same way you change tests in summary_factorlist(). Check the Help tab or online documentation for a reminder.

```
## group.1    1       1                911
## group.2    1       NA                18
##
##
##      Test of normality and Homoscedasticity:
##      -----------------------------------------
##
## Hawkins Test:
##
##      P-value for the Hawkins test of normality and homoscedasticity:  7.607252e-14
##
##    Either the test of multivariate normality or homoscedasticity (or both) is rejected.
##      Provided that normality can be assumed, the hypothesis of MCAR is
##      rejected at 0.05 significance level.
##
## Non-Parametric Test:
##
##      P-value for the non-parametric test of homoscedasticity:  0.6171955
##
##      Reject Normality at 0.05 significance level.
##      There is not sufficient evidence to reject MCAR at 0.05 significance level.
```

11.7   Handling missing data: MCAR

Prior to a standard regression analysis, we can either:

- Delete the variable with the missing data
- Delete the cases with the missing data
- Impute (fill in) the missing data
- Model the missing data

Using the examples, we identify that smoking (MCAR) is missing completely at random.

We know nothing about the missing values themselves, but we know of no plausible reason that the values of the missing data, for say, people who died should be different to the values of the missing data for those who survived. The pattern of missingness is therefore not felt to be MNAR.

11.7.1   Common solution: row-wise deletion

Depending on the number of data points that are missing, we may have sufficient power with complete cases to examine the relationships of interest.

We therefore elect to omit the patients in whom smoking is missing. This is known as list-wise deletion and will be performed by default and usually silently by any standard regression function.

```
explanatory <- c("age", "sex.factor",
                  "nodes", "obstruct.factor",
                  "smoking_mcar")
dependent <- "mort_5yr"
fit = colon_s %>%
  finalfit(dependent, explanatory)
```

TABLE 11.4: Regression analysis with missing data: List-wise deletion.

Dependent: Mortality 5 year		Alive	Died	OR (univariable)	OR (multivariable)
Age (years)	Mean (SD)	59.8 (11.4)	59.9 (12.5)	1.00 (0.99-1.01, p=0.986)	1.01 (1.00-1.02, p=0.200)
Sex	Female	243 (55.6)	194 (44.4)	-	-
	Male	268 (56.1)	210 (43.9)	0.98 (0.76-1.27, p=0.889)	1.02 (0.76-1.38, p=0.872)
nodes	Mean (SD)	2.7 (2.4)	4.9 (4.4)	1.24 (1.18-1.30, p<0.001)	1.25 (1.18-1.33, p<0.001)
Obstruction	No	408 (56.7)	312 (43.3)	-	-
	Yes	89 (51.1)	85 (48.9)	1.25 (0.90-1.74, p=0.189)	1.53 (1.05-2.22, p=0.027)
Smoking (MCAR)	Non-smoker	358 (56.4)	277 (43.6)	-	-
	Smoker	90 (49.7)	91 (50.3)	1.31 (0.94-1.82, p=0.113)	1.37 (0.96-1.96, p=0.083)

11.7.2   Other considerations

- Sensitivity analysis
- Omit the variable
- Imputation
- Model the missing data

If the variable in question is thought to be particularly important, you may wish to perform a sensitivity analysis. A sensitivity analysis in this context aims to capture the effect of uncertainty on the conclusions drawn from the model. Thus, you may choose to re-label all missing smoking values as "smoker", and see if that changes the conclusions of your analysis. The same procedure can be performed labelling with "non-smoker".

If smoking is not associated with the explanatory variable of interest or the outcome, it may be considered not to be a confounder and so could be omitted. That deals with the missing data issue, but of course may not always be appropriate.

Imputation and modelling are considered below.

11.8   Handling missing data: MAR

But life is rarely that simple.

Considering that the smoking variable is more likely to be missing if the patient is female (missing_compare shows a relationship). But, say, that the missing values are not different from the observed values. Missingness is then MAR.

If we simply drop all the patients for whom smoking is missing (list-wise deletion), then we drop relatively more females than men. This may have consequences for our conclusions if sex is associated with our explanatory variable of interest or outcome.

11.8.1   Common solution: Multivariate Imputation by Chained Equations (mice)

mice is our go to package for multiple imputation. That's the process of filling in missing data using a best-estimate from all the other data that exists. When first encountered, this may not sound like a good idea.

However, taking our simple example, if missingness in smoking is predicted strongly by sex (and other observed variables), and the values of the missing data are random, then we can impute (best-guess) the missing smoking values using sex and other variables in the dataset.

Imputation is not usually appropriate for the explanatory variable of interest or the outcome variable, although these can be used to impute other variables. In both cases, the hypothesis is that there is a meaningful association with other variables in the dataset, therefore it doesn't make sense to use these variables to impute them.

The process of multiple imputation involves:

*   **Impute** missing data m times, which results in m complete datasets
*   **Diagnose** the quality of the imputed values
*   **Analyse** each completed dataset
*   **Pool** the results of the repeated analyses

We will present a mice() example here. The package is well documented, and there are a number of checks and considerations that should be made to inform the imputation process. Read the documentation carefully prior to doing this yourself.

Note also missing_predictorMatrix() from **finalfit**. This provides a straightforward way to include or exclude variables to be imputed or to be used for imputation.

Impute

```
# Multivariate Imputation by Chained Equations (mice)
library(finalfit)
library(dplyr)
```

```
library(mice)
explanatory <- c("age", "sex.factor",
                 "nodes", "obstruct.factor", "smoking_mar")
dependent <- "mort_5yr"
```

Choose which variable to input missing values for and which variables to use
for the imputation process.

```
colon_s %>%
  select(dependent, explanatory) %>%
  missing_predictorMatrix(
    drop_from_imputed = c("obstruct.factor", "mort_5yr")
  ) -> predM
```

Make 10 imputed datasets and run our logistic regression analysis on each set.

```
fits <- colon_s %>%
  select(dependent, explanatory) %>%

  # Usually run imputation with 10 imputed sets, 4 here for demonstration
  mice(m = 4, predictorMatrix = predM) %>%

  # Run logistic regression on each imputed set
  with(glm(formula(ff_formula(dependent, explanatory)),
           family="binomial"))
```

```
##
## iter imp variable
##    1   1  mort_5yr  nodes  obstruct.factor  smoking_mar
##    1   2  mort_5yr  nodes  obstruct.factor  smoking_mar
##    1   3  mort_5yr  nodes  obstruct.factor  smoking_mar
##    1   4  mort_5yr  nodes  obstruct.factor  smoking_mar
##    2   1  mort_5yr  nodes  obstruct.factor  smoking_mar
##    2   2  mort_5yr  nodes  obstruct.factor  smoking_mar
##    2   3  mort_5yr  nodes  obstruct.factor  smoking_mar
##    2   4  mort_5yr  nodes  obstruct.factor  smoking_mar
##    3   1  mort_5yr  nodes  obstruct.factor  smoking_mar
##    3   2  mort_5yr  nodes  obstruct.factor  smoking_mar
##    3   3  mort_5yr  nodes  obstruct.factor  smoking_mar
##    3   4  mort_5yr  nodes  obstruct.factor  smoking_mar
##    4   1  mort_5yr  nodes  obstruct.factor  smoking_mar
##    4   2  mort_5yr  nodes  obstruct.factor  smoking_mar
##    4   3  mort_5yr  nodes  obstruct.factor  smoking_mar
##    4   4  mort_5yr  nodes  obstruct.factor  smoking_mar
##    5   1  mort_5yr  nodes  obstruct.factor  smoking_mar
##    5   2  mort_5yr  nodes  obstruct.factor  smoking_mar
##    5   3  mort_5yr  nodes  obstruct.factor  smoking_mar
##    5   4  mort_5yr  nodes  obstruct.factor  smoking_mar
```

Extract metrics from each model

```
# Examples of extracting metrics from fits and taking the mean
## AICs
fits %>%
  getfit() %>%
  purrr::map(AIC) %>%
  unlist() %>%
  mean()
```

```
## [1] 1193.679
```

```
# C-statistic
fits %>%
  getfit() %>%
  purrr::map(~ pROC::roc(.x$y, .x$fitted)$auc) %>%
  unlist() %>%
  mean()
```

```
## [1] 0.6789003
```

Pool models together

```
# Pool results
fits_pool <- fits %>%
  pool()
```

```
## Can be passed to or_plot
colon_s %>%
  or_plot(dependent, explanatory, glmfit = fits_pool, table_text_size=4)
```

Mortality 5 year: OR (95% CI, p-value)

Age (years)	-	1.01 (1.00-1.02, p=0.213)
Sex	Female	-
	Male	1.01 (0.77-1.34, p=0.924)
nodes	-	1.23 (1.17-1.29, p<0.001)
Obstruction	No	-
	Yes	1.34 (0.95-1.90, p=0.098)
Smoking (MAR)	Non-smoker	-
	Smoker	0.75 (0.50-1.14, p=0.178)

Odds ratio (95% CI, log scale)

```
# Summarise and put in table
fit_imputed <- fits_pool %>%
  fit2df(estimate_name = "OR (multiple imputation)", exp = TRUE)
```

```
# Use finalfit merge methods to create and compare results
explanatory <- c("age", "sex.factor",
                 "nodes", "obstruct.factor", "smoking_mar")
```

```
table_uni_multi <- colon_s %>%
  finalfit(dependent, explanatory, keep_fit_id = TRUE)

explanatory = c("age", "sex.factor",
                "nodes", "obstruct.factor")

fit_multi_no_smoking <- colon_s %>%
  glmmulti(dependent, explanatory) %>%
  fit2df(estimate_suffix = " (multivariable without smoking)")

# Combine to final table
table_imputed <-
  table_uni_multi %>%
  ff_merge(fit_multi_no_smoking) %>%
  ff_merge(fit_imputed, last_merge = TRUE)
```

TABLE 11.5: Regression analysis with missing data: Multiple imputation using mice().

Dependent: Mortality 5 year		Alive	Died	OR (univariable)	OR (multivariable)	OR (multivariable without smoking)	OR (multiple imputation)
Age (years)	Mean (SD)	59.8 (11.4)	59.9 (12.5)	1.00 (0.99-1.01, p=0.986)	1.02 (1.01-1.04, p=0.004)	1.01 (1.00-1.02, p=0.122)	1.01 (1.00-1.02, p=0.213)
Sex	Female	243 (55.6)	194 (44.4)	-	-	-	-
	Male	268 (56.1)	210 (43.9)	0.98 (0.76-1.27, p=0.889)	0.97 (0.69-1.34, p=0.836)	0.98 (0.74-1.30, p=0.890)	1.01 (0.77-1.34, p=0.924)
nodes	Mean (SD)	2.7 (2.4)	4.9 (4.4)	1.24 (1.18-1.30, p<0.001)	1.28 (1.21-1.37, p<0.001)	1.25 (1.19-1.32, p<0.001)	1.23 (1.17-1.29, p<0.001)
Obstruction	No	408 (56.7)	312 (43.3)	-	-	-	-
	Yes	89 (51.1)	85 (48.9)	1.25 (0.90-1.74, p=0.189)	1.49 (1.00-2.22, p=0.052)	1.36 (0.95-1.93, p=0.089)	1.34 (0.95-1.90, p=0.098)
Smoking (MAR)	Non-smoker	312 (54.0)	266 (46.0)				-
	Smoker	87 (62.6)	52 (37.4)	0.70 (0.48-1.02, p=0.067)	0.77 (0.51-1.16, p=0.221)	-	0.75 (0.50-1.14, p=0.178)

By examining the coefficients, the effect of the imputation compared with the complete case analysis can be seen.

Other considerations

- Omit the variable
- Model the missing data

As above, if the variable does not appear to be important, it may be omitted from the analysis. A sensitivity analysis in this context is another form of imputation. But rather than using all other available information to best-guess the missing data, we simply assign the value as above. Imputation is therefore likely to be more appropriate.

There is an alternative method to model the missing data for the categorical in this setting – just consider the missing data as a factor level. This has the advantage of simplicity, with the disadvantage of increasing the number of terms in the model.

```
library(dplyr)
explanatory = c("age", "sex.factor",
                "nodes", "obstruct.factor", "smoking_mar")
fit_explicit_na = colon_s %>%
  mutate(
    smoking_mar = forcats::fct_explicit_na(smoking_mar)
```

```
) %>%
finalfit(dependent, explanatory)
```

TABLE 11.6: Regression analysis with missing data: Explicitly modelling missing data.

Dependent: Mortality 5 year		Alive	Died	OR (univariable)	OR (multivariable)
Age (years)	Mean (SD)	59.8 (11.4)	59.9 (12.5)	1.00 (0.99-1.01, p=0.986)	1.01 (1.00-1.02, p=0.114)
Sex	Female	243 (55.6)	194 (44.4)	-	-
	Male	268 (56.1)	210 (43.9)	0.98 (0.76-1.27, p=0.889)	0.95 (0.71-1.28, p=0.743)
nodes	Mean (SD)	2.7 (2.4)	4.9 (4.4)	1.24 (1.18-1.30, p<0.001)	1.25 (1.19-1.32, p<0.001)
Obstruction	No	408 (56.7)	312 (43.3)	-	-
	Yes	89 (51.1)	85 (48.9)	1.25 (0.90-1.74, p=0.189)	1.35 (0.95-1.92, p=0.099)
Smoking (MAR)	Non-smoker	312 (54.0)	266 (46.0)	-	-
	Smoker	87 (62.6)	52 (37.4)	0.70 (0.48-1.02, p=0.067)	0.78 (0.52-1.17, p=0.233)
	(Missing)	112 (56.6)	86 (43.4)	0.90 (0.65-1.25, p=0.528)	0.85 (0.59-1.23, p=0.390)

11.9   Handling missing data: MNAR

Missing not at random data is tough in healthcare. To determine if data are MNAR for definite, we need to know their value in a subset of observations (patients).

Imagine that smoking status is poorly recorded in patients admitted to hospital as an emergency with an obstructing bowel cancer. Obstructing bowel cancers may be larger or their position may make the prognosis worse. Smoking may relate to the aggressiveness of the cancer and may be an independent predictor of prognosis. The missing values for smoking may therefore not be random. Smoking may be more common in the emergency patients and may be more common in those that die.

There is no easy way to handle this. If at all possible, try to get the missing data. Otherwise, be careful when drawing conclusions from analyses where data are thought to be missing not at random.

11.10   Summary

The more data analysis you do, the more you realise just how important missing data is. It is imperative that you understand where missing values exist in your own data. By following the simple steps in this chapter, you will be able to determine whether the cases (commonly patients) with missing values are a different population to those with complete data. This is the basis for understanding the impact of missing data on your analyses.

Whether you remove cases, remove variables, impute data, or model missing values, always check how each approach alters the conclusions of your analysis. Be transparent when you report your results and include the alternative approaches in appendices of published work.

12

Notebooks and Markdown

You ask me if I keep a notebook to record my great ideas. I've only ever had one.
Albert Einstein

12.1   What is a Notebook?

R is all-powerful for the manipulation, visualisation and analysis of data. What is often under-appreciated is the flexibility with which analyses can be exported or reported.

For instance, a full scientific paper, industry report, or monthly update can be easily written to accommodate a varying underlying dataset, and all tables and plots will be updated automatically.

This idea can be extended to a workflow in which all analyses are performed primarily within a document which doubles as the final report.

Enter "Data Notebooks"! Notebooks are documents which combine code and rich text elements, such as headings, paragraphs and links, in one document. They combine analysis and reporting in one human-readable document to provide an intuitive interface between the researcher and their analysis (Figure 12.1). This is sometimes called "literate programming", given the resulting logical structure of information can be easily read in the manner a human would read a book.

In our own work, we have now moved to doing most of our analyses in a Notebook file, rather than using a "script" file. You may not have guessed, but this whole book is written in this way.

Some of the advantages of the Notebook interface are:

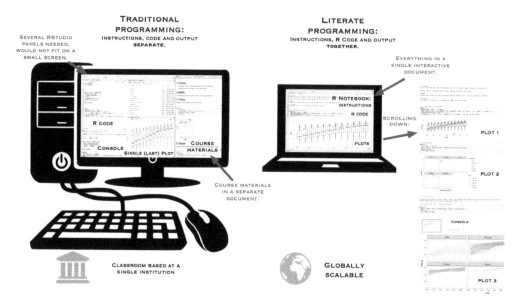

FIGURE 12.1: Traditional versus literate programming using Notebooks.

- code and output are adjacent to each other, so you are not constantly switching between "panes";
- easier to work on smaller screen, e.g., laptop;
- documentation and reporting can be done beside the code, text elements can be fully formatted;
- the code itself can be outputted or hidden;
- the code is not limited to R - you can use Python, SQL etc.;
- facilitate collaboration by easily sharing human-readable analysis documents;
- can be outputted in a number of formats including HTML (web page), PDF, and Microsoft Word;
- output can be extended to other formats such as presentations;
- training/learning may be easier as course materials, examples, and student notes are all in the same document.

12.2   What is Markdown?

Markdown is a lightweight language that can be used to write fully-formatted documents. It is plain-text and uses a simple set of rules to produce rather sophisticated output - we love it!

It is easy to format headings, bold text, italics, etc. Within RStudio there is a Quick Reference guide (Figure 12.2) and links to the RStudio cheatsheets[1] can be found in the Help drop-down menu.

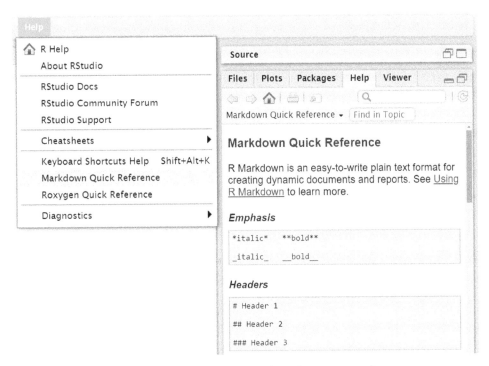

FIGURE 12.2: RStudio Markdown quick reference guide.

Markdown exists independent of R and is used by a range of techies and alike. A combination of Markdown (which is text with special characters to indicate desired formatting) and R code within it (usually to produce tables and plots) is called R Markdown. R scripts have the file extension .R, Markdown documents have a file extension .md, therefore, R Markdown documents are .Rmd.

12.3 What is the difference between a Notebook and an R Markdown file?

Most people use the terms R Notebook and R Markdown interchangeably and that is fine. Technically, R Markdown is a file, whereas R Notebook is a way to work with R Markdown files. R Notebooks do not have their own file format, they all use .Rmd. All R Notebooks can be 'knitted' to R Markdown outputs, and all R Markdown documents can be interfaced as a Notebook.

[1] https://www.rstudio.com/resources/cheatsheets

An important difference is in the execution of code. In R Markdown, when the file is Knit, all the elements (chunks) are also run. Knit is to R Markdown what Source is to an R script (Source was introduced in Chapter 1, essentially it means 'Run all lines').

In a Notebook, when the file is rendered with the Preview button, no code is re-run, only that which has already been run and is present in the document is included in the output. Also, in the Notebook behind-the-scenes file (.nb), all the code is always included. Something to watch out for if your code contains sensitive information, such as a password (which it never should!).

12.4   Notebook vs HTML vs PDF vs Word

In RStudio, a Notebook can be created by going to:
File -> New File -> R Notebook

Alternatively, you can create a Markdown file using:
File -> New File -> R Markdown...

Don't worry which you choose. As mentioned above, they are essentially the same thing but just come with different options. It is easy to switch from a Notebook to a Markdown file if you wish to create a PDF or Word document for instance.

If you are primarily doing analysis in the Notebook environment, choose Notebook. If you are primarily creating a PDF or Word document, choose R Markdown file.

12.5   The anatomy of a Notebook / R Markdown file

When you create a file, a helpful template is provided to get you started. Figure 12.3 shows the essential elements of a Notebook file and how these translate to the HTML preview.

12.5.1   YAML header

Every Notebook and Markdown file requires a "YAML header". Where do they get these terms you ask? Originally YAML was said to mean Yet Another Markup Language, referencing its purpose as a markup language. It was later repurposed as YAML Ain't Markup Language, a recursive acronym, to distinguish its purpose as data-oriented rather than document markup (thank you Wikipedia).

This is simply where many of the settings/options for file creation are placed. In RStudio, these often update automatically as different settings are invoked in the Options menu.

12.5.2 R code chunks

R code within a Notebook or Markdown file can be included in two ways:

- in-line: e.g., the total number of oranges was `` `r sum(fruit$oranges)` ``;
- as a "chunk".

R chunks are flexible, come with lots of options, and you will soon get into the way of using them.

Figure 12.3 shows how a chunk fits into the document.

```{r}
# This is basic chunk.
# It always starts with ```{r}
# And ends with ```
# Code goes here
sum(fruit$oranges)
```

This may look off-putting, but just go with it for now. You can type the four back-ticks in manually, or use the Insert button and choose R. You will also notice that chunks are not limited to R code. It is particularly helpful that Python can also be run in this way.

When doing an analysis in a Notebook you will almost always want to see the code and the output. When you are creating a final document you may wish to hide code. Chunk behaviour can be controlled via the Chunk Cog on the right of the chunk (Figure 12.3).

Table 12.1 shows the various permutations of code and output options that are available. The code is placed in the chunk header but the options fly-out now does this automatically, e.g.,

```{r, echo=FALSE}
```

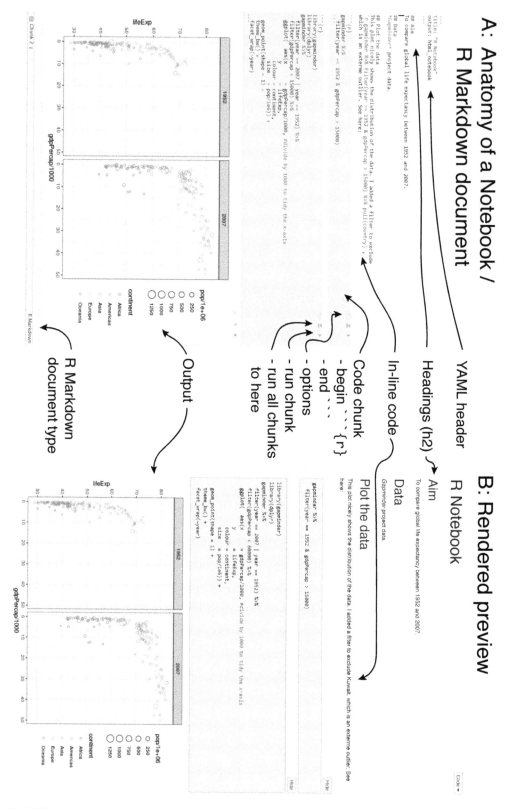

FIGURE 12.3: The Anatomy of a Notebook/Markdown file. Input (left) and output (right).

TABLE 12.1: Chunk output options when knitting an R Markdown file. When using the Chunk Cog, RStudio will add these options appropriately; there is no need to memorise them.

Option	Code
Show output only	echo=FALSE
Show code and output	echo=TRUE
Show code (don't run code)	eval=FALSE
Show nothing (run code)	include=FALSE
Show nothing (don't run code)	include=FALSE, eval=FALSE
Hide warnings	warnings=FALSE
Hide messages	messages=FALSE

12.5.3 Setting default chunk options

We can set default options for all our chunks at the top of our document by adding and editing `knitr::opts_chunk$set(echo = TRUE)` at the top of the document.

```{r}
knitr::opts_chunk$set(echo = TRUE,
                      warning = FALSE)
```

12.5.4 Setting default figure options

It is possible to set different default sizes for different output types by including these in the YAML header (or using the document cog):

```
---
title: "R Notebook"
output:
  pdf_document:
    fig_height: 3
    fig_width: 4
  html_document:
    fig_height: 6
    fig_width: 9
---
```

The YAML header is very sensitive to the spaces/tabs, so make sure these are correct.

12.5.5 Markdown elements

Markdown text can be included as you wish around your chunks. Figure 12.3 shows an example of how this can be done. This is a great way of getting into the habit of explicitly documenting your analysis. When you come back to a file in 6 months' time, all of your thinking is there in front of you, rather than having to work out what on Earth you were on about from a collection of random code!

12.6 Interface and outputting

12.6.1 Running code and chunks, knitting

Figure 12.4 shows the various controls for running chunks and producing an output document. Code can be run line-by-line using `Ctrl+Enter` as you are used to. There are options for running all the chunks above the current chunk you are working on. This is useful as a chunk you are working on will often rely on objects created in preceding chunks.

It is good practice to use the `Restart R` and `Run All Chunks` option in the `Run` menu every so often. This ensures that all the code in your document is self-contained and is not relying on an object in the environment which you have created elsewhere. If this was the case, it will fail when rendering a Markdown document.

Probably the most important engine behind the RStudio Notebooks functionality is the **knitr** package by Yihui Xie.

Not knitting like your granny does, but rendering a Markdown document into an output file, such as HTML, PDF or Word. There are many options which can be applied in order to achieve the desired output. Some of these have been specifically coded into RStudio (Figure 12.4).

PDF document creation requires a `LaTex` distribution to be installed on your computer. Depending on what system you are using, this may be setup already. An easy way to do this is using the **tinytex** package.

```{r}
install.packages("tinytex")
# Restart R, then run
tinytex::install_tinytex()
```

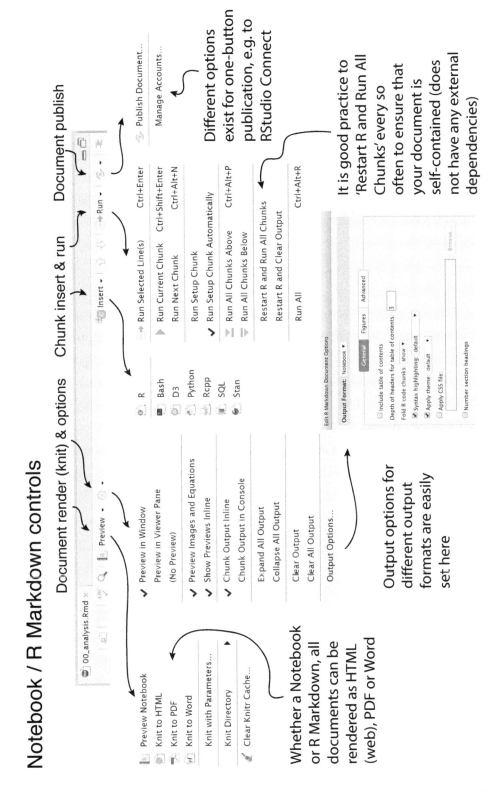

FIGURE 12.4: Chunk and document options in Notebook/Markdown files.

In the next chapter we will focus on the details of producing a polished final document.

12.7   File structure and workflow

As projects get bigger, it is important that they are well organised. This will avoid errors and make collaboration easier.

What is absolutely compulsory is that your analysis must reside within an RStudio Project and have a meaningful name (not MyProject! or Analysis1). Creating a New Project on RStudio will automatically create a new folder for itself (unless you choose "Existing Folder"). Never work within a generic Home or Documents directory. Furthermore, do not change the working directory using `setwd()` - there is no reason to do this, and it usually makes your analysis less reproducible. Once you're starting to get the hang of R, you should initiate all Projects with a Git repository for version control (see Chapter 13).

For smaller projects with 1-2 data files, a couple of scripts and an R Markdown document, it is fine to keep them all in the Project folder (but we repeat, each Project must have its own folder). Once the number of files grows beyond that, you should add separate folders for different types of files.

Here is our suggested approach. Based on the nature of your analyses, the number of folders may be smaller or greater than this, and they may be called something different.

```
proj/
- scripts/
- data_raw/
- data_processed/
- figures/
- 00_analysis.Rmd
```

`scripts/` contains all the `.R` script files used for data cleaning/preparation. If you only have a few scripts, it's fine to not have this one and just keep the `.R` files in the project folder (where `00_analysis.Rmd` is in the above example). `data_raw/` contains all raw data, such as `.csv` files, `data_processed/` contains data you've taken from raw, cleaned, modified, joined or otherwise changed using R scripts. `figures/` may contain plots (e.g., `.png`, `.jpg`, `.pdf`) `00_analysis.Rmd` or `00_analysis.R` is the actual main working file, and we keep this in the main project directory.

Your R scripts should be numbered using double digits, and they should have meaningful names, for example:

```
scripts/00_source_all.R
scripts/01_read_data.R
scripts/02_make_factors.R
scripts/03_duplicate_records.R
```

For instance, `01_read_data.R` may look like this.

```
# Melanoma project
## Data pull

# Get data
library(readr)
melanoma <- read_csv(
  here::here("data_raw", "melanoma.csv")
)

# Other basic reccoding or renaming functions here

# Save
save(melanoma, file =
  here::here("data_processed", "melanoma_working.rda")
)
```

Note the use of `here::here()`. RStudio projects manage working directories in a better way than `setwd()`. `here::here()` is useful when sharing projects between Linux, Mac and Windows machines, which have different conventions for file paths.

For instance, on a Mac you would otherwise do `read_csv("data/melanoma.csv")` and on Windows you would have to do `read_csv("data\melanoma.csv")`. Having to include either / (GNU/Linux, macOS) or \ (Windows) in your script means it will have to be changed by hand when running on a different system. What `here::here("data_raw", "melanoma.csv")`, however, works on any system, as it will use an appropriate one 'behind the scenes' without you having to change anything.

`02_make_factors.R` is our example second file, but it could be anything you want. It could look something like this.

```
# Melanoma project
## Create factors
library(tidyverse)

load(
  here::here("data_processed", "melanoma_working.rda")
)

## Recode variables
melanoma <- melanoma %>%
  mutate(
    sex = factor(sex) %>%
      fct_recode("Male" = "1",
```

```
              "Female" = "0")
  )

# Save
save(melanoma, file =
  here::here("data", "melanoma_working.rda")
)
```

All these files can then be brought together in a single file to `source()`. This function is used to run code from a file.

`00_source_all.R` might look like this:

```
# Melanoma project
## Source all

source( here::here("scripts", "01_data_upload.R") )
source( here::here("scripts", "02_make_factors.R") )
source( here::here("scripts", "03_duplicate_records.R") )

# Save
save(melanoma, file =
  here::here("data_processed", "melanoma_final.rda")
)
```

You can now bring your robustly prepared data into your analysis file, which can be `.R` or `.Rmd` if you are working in a Notebook. We call this `00_analysis.Rmd` and it always sits in the project root director. You have two options in bringing in the data.

1. `source("00_source_all.R")` to re-load and process the data again
    - this is useful if the data is changing
    - may take a long time if it is a large dataset with lots of manipulations
2. `load("melanoma_final.rda")` from the `data_processed/` folder
    - usually quicker, but loads the dataset which was created the last time you ran `00_source_all.R`

Remember: For `.R` files use `source()`, for `.rda` files use `load()`.

The two options look like this:

```
---
title: "Melanoma analysis"
output: html_notebook
---

```{r get-data-option-1, echo=FALSE}
load(
  here:here("data", "melanoma_all.rda")
)
```

```{r get-data-option-2, echo=FALSE}
source(
  here:here("R", "00_source_all.R")
)
```

12.7.1 Why go to all this bother?

It comes from many years of finding errors due to badly organised projects. It is not needed for a small quick project, but is essential for any major work.

At the very start of an analysis (as in the first day), we will start working in a single file. We will quickly move chunks of data cleaning / preparation code into separate files as we go.

Compartmentalising the data cleaning helps with finding and dealing with errors ('debugging'). Sourced files can be 'commented out' (adding a # to a line in the `00_source_all.R` file) if you wish to exclude the manipulations in that particular file.

Most important, it helps with collaboration. When multiple people are working on a project, it is essential that communication is good and everybody is working to the same overall plan.
```

13

Exporting and reporting

Without data, you are just another person with an opinion.
W. Edwards Deming

The results of any data analysis are meaningless if they are not effectively communicated.

This may be as a journal article or presentation, or perhaps a regular report or webpage. In Chapter 13 we emphasise another of the major strengths of R - the ease with which HTML (a web page), PDF, or Word documents can be generated.

The purpose of this chapter is to focus on the details of how to get your exported tables, plots and documents looking exactly the way you want them. There are many customisations that can be used, and we will only touch on a few of these.

We will generate a report using data already familiar to you from this book. It will contain two tables - a demographics table and a regression table - and a plot. We will use the `colon_s` data from the `finalfit` package. What follows is for demonstration purposes and is not meant to illustrate model building. For the purposes of the demonstration, we will ask, does a particular characteristic of a colon cancer (e.g., cancer differentiation) predict 5-year survival?

13.1 Which format should I use?

The three common formats for exporting reports have different pros and cons:

- HTML is the least fussy to work with and can resize itself and its content automatically. For rapid exploration and prototyping, we recommend knitting to HTML. HTML documents can be attached to emails and viewed using any browser, even with no internet access (as long as it is a self-contained HTML document, which R Markdown exports usually are).

- PDF looks most professional when printed. This is because R Markdown uses LaTeX to typeset PDF documents. LaTeX PDFs are our preferred method of producing printable reports or dissertations, but they come with their own bag of issues. Mainly that LaTeX figures and tables *float* and may therefore appear much later down the document than the original text describing it was.
- Word is useful when working with non-R people who need to edit your output.

13.2   Working in a .r file

We will demonstrate how you might put together a report in two ways.

First, we will show what you might do if you were working in standard R script file, then exporting certain objects only.

Second, we will talk about the approach if you were primarily working in a Notebook, which makes things easier.

We presume that the data have been cleaned carefully and the 'Get the data', 'Check the data', 'Data exploration' and 'Model building' steps have already been completed.

13.3   Demographics table

First, let's look at associations between our explanatory variable of interest (exposure) and other explanatory variables.

```r
library(tidyverse)
library(finalfit)

# Specify explanatory variables of interest
explanatory <- c("age", "sex.factor",
                "extent.factor", "obstruct.factor",
                "nodes")

colon_s %>%
```

```
summary_factorlist("differ.factor", explanatory,
                   p=TRUE, na_include=TRUE)
```

TABLE 13.1: Exporting 'table 1': Tumour differentiation by patient and disease factors.

label	levels	Well	Moderate	Poor	p
Age (years)	Mean (SD)	60.2 (12.8)	59.9 (11.7)	59.0 (12.8)	0.644
Sex	Female	51 (54.8)	314 (47.4)	73 (48.7)	0.400
	Male	42 (45.2)	349 (52.6)	77 (51.3)	
Extent of spread	Submucosa	5 (5.4)	12 (1.8)	3 (2.0)	0.081
	Muscle	12 (12.9)	78 (11.8)	12 (8.0)	
	Serosa	76 (81.7)	542 (81.7)	127 (84.7)	
	Adjacent structures	0 (0.0)	31 (4.7)	8 (5.3)	
Obstruction	No	69 (74.2)	531 (80.1)	114 (76.0)	0.655
	Yes	19 (20.4)	122 (18.4)	31 (20.7)	
	(Missing)	5 (5.4)	10 (1.5)	5 (3.3)	
nodes	Mean (SD)	2.7 (2.2)	3.6 (3.4)	4.7 (4.4)	<0.001

Note that we include missing data in this table (see Chapter 11).

Also note that nodes has not been labelled properly.

In addition, there are small numbers in some variables generating chisq.test() warnings (expect fewer than 5 in any cell).

Now generate a final table.[1]

```
colon_s <- colon_s %>%
  mutate(
    nodes = ff_label(nodes, "Lymph nodes involved")
    )

table1 <- colon_s %>%
  summary_factorlist("differ.factor", explanatory,
                     p=TRUE, na_include=TRUE,
                     add_dependent_label=TRUE,
                     dependent_label_prefix = "Exposure: "
                     )
table1
```

---

[1]The finalfit functions used here - summary_factorlist() and finalfit() were introduced in Part II - Data Analysis. We will therefore not describe the different arguments here, we use them to demonstrate R's powers of exporting to fully formatted output documents.

TABLE 13.2: Exporting table 1: Adjusting labels and output.

Exposure: Differentiation		Well	Moderate	Poor	p
Age (years)	Mean (SD)	60.2 (12.8)	59.9 (11.7)	59.0 (12.8)	0.644
Sex	Female	51 (54.8)	314 (47.4)	73 (48.7)	0.400
	Male	42 (45.2)	349 (52.6)	77 (51.3)	
Extent of spread	Submucosa	5 (5.4)	12 (1.8)	3 (2.0)	0.081
	Muscle	12 (12.9)	78 (11.8)	12 (8.0)	
	Serosa	76 (81.7)	542 (81.7)	127 (84.7)	
	Adjacent structures	0 (0.0)	31 (4.7)	8 (5.3)	
Obstruction	No	69 (74.2)	531 (80.1)	114 (76.0)	0.655
	Yes	19 (20.4)	122 (18.4)	31 (20.7)	
	(Missing)	5 (5.4)	10 (1.5)	5 (3.3)	
Lymph nodes involved	Mean (SD)	2.7 (2.2)	3.6 (3.4)	4.7 (4.4)	<0.001

13.4 Logistic regression table

After investigating the relationships between our explanatory variables, we will use logistic regression to include the outcome variable.

```
explanatory <- c( "differ.factor", "age", "sex.factor",
            "extent.factor", "obstruct.factor",
            "nodes")
dependent <- "mort_5yr"
table2 <- colon_s %>%
  finalfit(dependent, explanatory,
        dependent_label_prefix = "")
table2
```

TABLE 13.3: Exporting a regression results table.

Mortality 5 year		Alive	Died	OR (univariable)	OR (multivariable)
Differentiation	Well	52 (56.5)	40 (43.5)	-	-
	Moderate	382 (58.7)	269 (41.3)	0.92 (0.59-1.43, p=0.694)	0.62 (0.38-1.01, p=0.054)
	Poor	63 (42.3)	86 (57.7)	1.77 (1.05-3.01, p=0.032)	1.00 (0.56-1.78, p=0.988)
Age (years)	Mean (SD)	59.8 (11.4)	59.9 (12.5)	1.00 (0.99-1.01, p=0.986)	1.01 (1.00-1.02, p=0.098)
Sex	Female	243 (55.6)	194 (44.4)	-	-
	Male	268 (56.1)	210 (43.9)	0.98 (0.76-1.27, p=0.889)	0.97 (0.73-1.30, p=0.858)
Extent of spread	Submucosa	16 (80.0)	4 (20.0)	-	-
	Muscle	78 (75.7)	25 (24.3)	1.28 (0.42-4.79, p=0.681)	1.25 (0.36-5.87, p=0.742)
	Serosa	401 (53.5)	349 (46.5)	3.48 (1.26-12.24, p=0.027)	3.03 (0.96-13.36, p=0.087)
	Adjacent structures	16 (38.1)	26 (61.9)	6.50 (1.98-25.93, p=0.004)	6.80 (1.75-34.55, p=0.010)
Obstruction	No	408 (56.7)	312 (43.3)	-	-
	Yes	89 (51.1)	85 (48.9)	1.25 (0.90-1.74, p=0.189)	1.26 (0.88-1.82, p=0.206)
Lymph nodes involved	Mean (SD)	2.7 (2.4)	4.9 (4.4)	1.24 (1.18-1.30, p<0.001)	1.24 (1.18-1.31, p<0.001)

13.5 Odds ratio plot

It is often preferable to express the coefficients from a regression model as a forest plot. For instance, a plot of odds ratios can be produced using the or_plot() function also from the finalfit package:

```
colon_s %>%
  or_plot(dependent, explanatory,
          breaks = c(0.5, 1, 5, 10, 20, 30),
          table_text_size = 3.5)
```

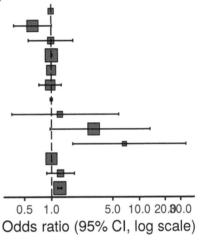

Mortality 5 year: OR (95% CI, p-value)

Differentiation	Well	-
	Moderate	0.62 (0.38-1.01, p=0.054)
	Poor	1.00 (0.56-1.78, p=0.988)
Age (years)	-	1.01 (1.00-1.02, p=0.098)
Sex	Female	-
	Male	0.97 (0.73-1.30, p=0.858)
Extent of spread	Submucosa	-
	Muscle	1.25 (0.36-5.87, p=0.742)
	Serosa	3.03 (0.96-13.36, p=0.087)
	Adjacent structures	6.80 (1.75-34.55, p=0.010)
Obstruction	No	-
	Yes	1.26 (0.88-1.82, p=0.206)
Lymph nodes involved	-	1.24 (1.18-1.31, p<0.001)

Odds ratio (95% CI, log scale)

FIGURE 13.1: Odds ratio plot.

13.6 MS Word via knitr/R Markdown

When moving from a .r file to a Markdown (.Rmd) file, environment objects such as tables or data frames / tibbles usually require to be saved and loaded to R Markdown document.

```
# Save objects for knitr/markdown
save(table1, table2, dependent, explanatory,
     file = here::here("data", "out.rda"))
```

In RStudio, select:
File > New File > R Markdown

A useful template file is produced by default. Try hitting knit to Word on the Knit button at the top of the `.Rmd` script window. If you have difficulties at this stage, refer to Chapter 12.

Now paste this into the file (we'll call it Example 1):

```
---
title: "Example knitr/R Markdown document"
author: "Your name"
date: "22/5/2020"
output:
  word_document: default
---

```{r setup, include=FALSE}
# Load data into global environment.
library(finalfit)
library(dplyr)
library(knitr)
load(here::here("data", "out.rda"))
```

Table 1 - Demographics
```{r table1, echo = FALSE}
kable(table1, row.names=FALSE, align=c("l", "l", "r", "r", "r", "r"))
```

Table 2 - Association between tumour factors and 5 year mortality
```{r table2, echo = FALSE}
kable(table2, row.names=FALSE, align=c("l", "l", "r", "r", "r", "r"))
```

Figure 1 - Association between tumour factors and 5 year mortality
```{r figure1, echo = FALSE}
explanatory = c( "differ.factor", "age", "sex.factor",
                "extent.factor", "obstruct.factor",
                "nodes")
dependent = "mort_5yr"
colon_s %>%
  or_plot(dependent, explanatory)
```
```

Knitting this into a Word document results in Figure 13.2A), which looks pretty decent but some of the columns need some formatting and the plot needs resized. Do not be tempted to do this by hand directly in the Word document.

Yes, before Markdown, we would have to move and format each table and figure directly in Word, and we would repeat this every time something changed. Turns out some patient records were duplicated and you have to remove them

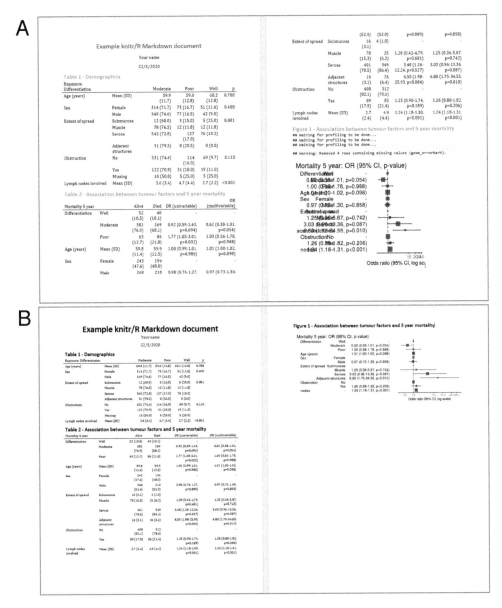

FIGURE 13.2: Knitting to Microsoft Word from R Markdown. Before (A) and after (B) adjustment.

before repeating the analysis over again. Or your colleague forgot to attach an extra file with 10 more patients.

No problem, you update the dataset, re-run the script that created the tables and hit Knit in the R Markdown document. No more mindless re-doing for you. We think this is pretty amazing.

13.6.1 Figure quality in Word output

If your plots are looking a bit grainy in Word, include this in your setup chunk for high quality:

```
knitr::opts_chunk$set(dpi = 300)
```

The setup chunk is the one that starts with ```` ```{r setup, include = FALSE} ```` and is generated automatically when you create a new R Markdown document in RStudio.

13.7 Create Word template file

To make sure tables always export with a suitable font size, you may edit your Word file but only to create a new template. You will then use this template to Knit the R Markdown document again.

In the Word document the first example outputted, click on a table. The style should be `compact`: Right-click > Modify... > font size = 9

Alter heading and text styles in the same way as desired. Save this as `colon-Template.docx` (avoid underscores in the name of this file). Move the file to your project folder and reference it in your `.Rmd` YAML header, as shown below. Make sure you get the spacing correct, unlike R code, the YAML header is sensitive to formatting and the number of spaces at the beginning of the argument lines.

Finally, to get the figure printed in a size where the labels don't overlap each other, you will have to specify a width for it. The Chunk cog introduced in the previous chapter is a convenient way to change the figure size (it is in the top-right corner of each grey code chunk in an R Markdown document). It usually takes some experimentation to find the best size for each plot/output document; in this case we are going with `fig.width = 10`.

Knitting Example 2 here gives us Figure 13.2B). For something that is generated automatically, it looks awesome.

```
---
title: "Example knitr/R Markdown document"
author: "Your name"
date: "22/5/2020"
output:
  word_document:
    reference_docx: colonTemplate.docx
---

```{r setup, include=FALSE}
# Load data into global environment.
library(finalfit)
library(dplyr)
library(knitr)
load(here::here("data", "out.rda"))
```

Table 1 - Demographics
```{r table1, echo = FALSE}
kable(table1, row.names=FALSE, align=c("l", "l", "r", "r", "r", "r"))
```

Table 2 - Association between tumour factors and 5 year mortality
```{r table2, echo = FALSE}
kable(table2, row.names=FALSE, align=c("l", "l", "r", "r", "r", "r"))
```

Figure 1 - Association between tumour factors and 5 year mortality
```{r figure1, echo=FALSE, message=FALSE, warning=FALSE, fig.width=10}
explanatory = c( "differ.factor", "age", "sex.factor",
                 "extent.factor", "obstruct.factor",
                 "nodes")
dependent = "mort_5yr"
colon_s %>%
  or_plot(dependent, explanatory,
          breaks = c(0.5, 1, 5, 10, 20, 30))
```
```

13.8 PDF via knitr/R Markdown

Without changing anything in Example 1 and Knitting it into a PDF, we get 13.3A.

Again, most of it already looks pretty good, but some parts over-run the page and the plot is not a good size.

We can fix the plot in exactly the same way we did for the Word version (`fig.width`), but the second table that is too wide needs some special handling.

For this we use `kable_styling(font_size=8)` from the `kableExtra` package. Remember to install it when using for the first time, and include `library(knitExtra)` alongside the other library lines at the setup chunk.

We will also alter the margins of your page using the geometry option in the preamble as the default margins of a PDF document coming out of R Markdown are a bit wide for us.

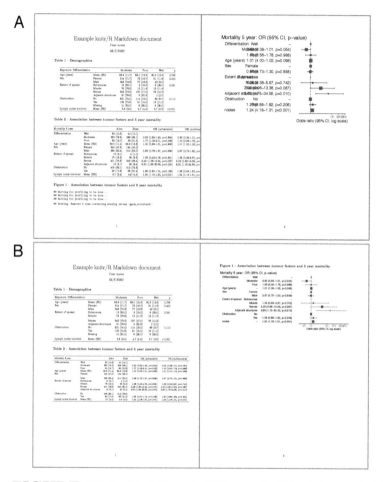

FIGURE 13.3: Knitting to Microsoft Word from R Markdown. Before (A) and after (B) adjustment.

```
---
title: "Example knitr/R Markdown document"
author: "Your name"
date: "22/5/2020"
output:
  pdf_document: default
geometry: margin=0.75in
---
```

```
```{r setup, include=FALSE}
# Load data into global environment.
library(finalfit)
library(dplyr)
library(knitr)
library(kableExtra)
load(here::here("data", "out.rda"))
```

Table 1 - Demographics
```{r table1, echo = FALSE}
kable(table1, row.names=FALSE, align=c("l", "l", "r", "r", "r", "r"),
      booktabs = TRUE)
```

Table 2 - Association between tumour factors and 5 year mortality
```{r table2, echo = FALSE}
kable(table2, row.names=FALSE, align=c("l", "l", "r", "r", "r", "r"),
      booktabs=TRUE) %>%
kable_styling(font_size=8)
```

Figure 1 - Association between tumour factors and 5 year mortality
```{r figure1, echo=FALSE, message=FALSE, warning=FALSE, fig.width=10}
explanatory = c( "differ.factor", "age", "sex.factor",
                 "extent.factor", "obstruct.factor",
                 "nodes")
dependent = "mort_5yr"
colon_s %>%
  or_plot(dependent, explanatory,
          breaks = c(0.5, 1, 5, 10, 20, 30))
```
```

The result is shown in Figure 13.3B.

13.9 Working in a .Rmd file

We now perform almost all our analyses in a Notebook / Markdown file as described in the previous chapter. This means running all analyses within the document, without the requirement to save and reload table or plot objects.

As mentioned earlier, a Notebook document can be rendered as a PDF or a Word document. Some refining is usually needed to move from an 'analysis' document to a final 'report' document, but it is often minimal.

Figure 13.4 demonstrates a report-type document rendered as a PDF. All the code is run within the document, but not included in the output (echo=FALSE).

Outcomes after resection for colorectal cancer

The Colorectal Cancer Collaborative

Introduction

Colorectal cancer is the third most common cancer worldwide. In this study, we have re-analysed a classic dataset to determine the influence of tumour differentiation on 5-year survival prior to the introduction of modern chemotherapeutic regimes.

Methods

Data were generated within a randomised trial of adjuvant chemotherapy for colon cancer. Levamisole is a low-toxicity compound etc. etc.

Results

Patient characteristics

Table 1 shows the characteristics of patients in the study.

Table 1: Demographics of patients entered into randomised controlled trial of adjuvant chemotherapy after surgery for colon cancer.

Exposure: Differentiation		Moderate	Poor	Well	p
Age (years)	Mean (SD)	59.9 (11.7)	59.0 (12.8)	60.2 (12.8)	0.788
Sex	Female	314 (71.7)	73 (16.7)	51 (11.6)	0.400
	Male	349 (74.6)	77 (16.5)	42 (9.0)	
Extent of spread	Submucosa	12 (60.0)	3 (15.0)	5 (25.0)	0.081
	Muscle	78 (76.5)	12 (11.8)	12 (11.8)	
	Serosa	542 (72.8)	127 (17.0)	76 (10.2)	
	Adjacent structures	31 (79.5)	8 (20.5)	0 (0.0)	
Lymph nodes involved	Mean (SD)	3.6 (3.4)	4.7 (4.4)	2.7 (2.2)	<0.001

5-year outcome by tumour differentiation

Table 2 shows a univariable and multivariable regression analysis of 5-year mortality by patient and disease characteristics.

Table 2: 5-year survival after colon cancer (logistic regression)

Mortality 5 year		Alive	Died	OR (univariable)	OR (multivariable)
Differentiation	Well	52 (10.5)	40 (10.1)	-	-
	Moderate	382 (76.9)	269 (68.1)	0.92 (0.59-1.43, p=0.694)	0.70 (0.44-1.12, p=0.132)
	Poor	63 (12.7)	86 (21.8)	1.77 (1.05-3.01, p=0.032)	1.08 (0.61-1.90, p=0.796)
Age (years)	Mean (SD)	59.8 (11.4)	59.9 (12.5)	1.00 (0.99-1.01, p=0.986)	1.01 (1.00-1.02, p=0.195)
Sex	Female	243 (47.6)	194 (48.0)	-	-
	Male	268 (52.4)	210 (52.0)	0.98 (0.76-1.27, p=0.889)	0.98 (0.74-1.30, p=0.885)
Extent of spread	Submucosa	16 (3.1)	4 (1.0)	-	-
	Muscle	78 (15.3)	25 (6.2)	1.28 (0.42-4.79, p=0.681)	1.28 (0.37-5.92, p=0.722)
	Serosa	401 (78.5)	349 (86.4)	3.48 (1.26-12.24, p=0.027)	3.13 (1.01-13.76, p=0.076)
	Adjacent structures	16 (3.1)	26 (6.4)	6.50 (1.98-25.93, p=0.004)	6.04 (1.58-30.41, p=0.015)
Lymph nodes involved	Mean (SD)	2.7 (2.4)	4.9 (4.4)	1.24 (1.18-1.30, p<0.001)	1.23 (1.17-1.30, p<0.001)

Discussion

In this study etc.

1

FIGURE 13.4: Writing a final report in a Markdown document.

13.10   Moving between formats

As we have shown, it is relatively straightforward to move between HTML, Word and PDF when documents are simple. This becomes more difficult if you have a complicated document which includes lots of formatting.

For instance, if you use the package `kableExtra()` to customise your tables, you can only export to HTML and PDF. Knitting to Word will not currently work with advanced `kableExtra` functions in your R Markdown document. Similarly, `flextable` and `officer` are excellent packages for a love story between R Markdown and Word/MS Office, but they do not work for HTML or PDF.

13.11   Summary

The combination of R, RStudio, and Markdown is a powerful triumvirate which produces beautiful results quickly and will be greatly labour saving. We use this combination for all academic work, but also in the production of real-time reports such as webpages and downloadable PDFs for ongoing projects. This is a fast-moving area with new applications and features appearing every month. We would highly recommend you spend some time getting familiar with this area, as it will become an ever more important skill in the future.

14

Version control

Version control is essential for keeping track of data analysis projects, as well as collaborating. It allows backup of scripts and collaboration on complex projects. RStudio works really well with Git, an open source distributed version control system, and GitHub, a web-based Git repository hosting service.

Git is a piece of software which runs locally. It may need to be installed first.

It is important to highlight the difference between Git (local version control software) and GitHub (a web-based repository store).

14.1 Setup Git on RStudio and associate with GitHub

In RStudio, go to Tools -> Global Options and select the **Git/SVN** tab. Ensure the path to the Git executable is correct. This is particularly impor tant in Windows where it may not default correctly (e.g., `C:/Program Files (x86)/Git/bin/git.exe`).

14.2 Create an SSH RSA key and add to your GitHub account

In the **Git/SVN** tab, hit *Create RSA Key* (Figure 14.1A). In the window that appears, hit the *Create* button (Figure 14.1B). Close this window.

Click, *View public key* (Figure 14.1C), and copy the displayed public key (Figure 14.1D).

If you haven't already, create a GitHub account. On the GitHub website, open the account settings tab and click the SSH keys tab (Figure 14.2A). Click *Add SSH key* and paste in the public key you have copied from RStudio Figure 14.2B).

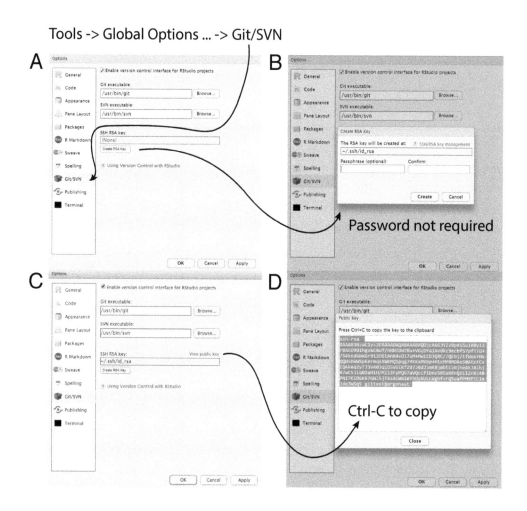

FIGURE 14.1: Creating an SSH key in RStudio's Global Options.

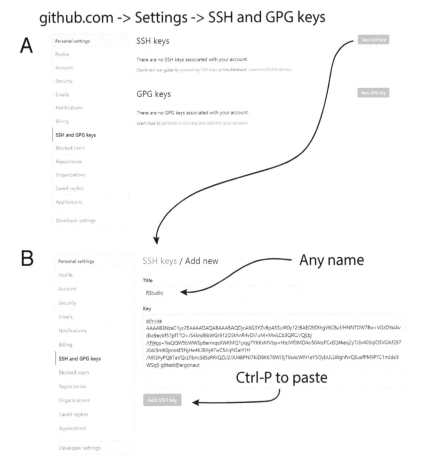

FIGURE 14.2: Adding your RStudio SSH key to your GitHub account.

14.3 Create a project in RStudio and commit a file

Next, return to RStudio and configure Git via the **Terminal** (Figure 14.3A)). Remember Git is a piece of software running on your own computer. This is distinct to GitHub, which is the repository website.

We will now create a new project which we want to backup to GitHub.

In RStudio, click *New project* as normal (Figure 14.3B). Click *New Directory*. Name the project and check *Create a git repository*. Now in RStudio, create a new script which you will add to your repository.

After saving your new script (e.g., test.R), it should appear in the **Git** tab beside **Environment**.

Tick the file you wish to add, and the status should turn to a green 'A' (Figure 14.3C). Now click *Commit* and enter an identifying message in Commit message (Figure 14.3D). It makes sense to do this prior to linking the project and the GitHub repository, otherwise you'll have nothing to push to GitHub.

You have now committed the current version of this file to a Git repository on your computer/server.

14.4   Create a new repository on GitHub and link to RStudio project

Now you may want to push the contents of this commit to GitHub, so it is also backed-up off site and available to collaborators. As always, you must exercise caution when working with sensitive data. Take steps to stop yourself from accidentally pushing whole datasets to GitHub.[1] You only want to push R code to GitHub, not the (sensitive) data.

When you see a dataset appear in the Git tab of your RStudio, select it, then click on More, and then Ignore. This means the file does not get included in your Git repository, and it does not get pushed to GitHub. GitHub is not for backing up sensitive datasets, it's for backing up R code. And make sure your R code does not include passwords or access tokens.

In GitHub, create a *New repository*, called here myproject (Figure 14.4A). You will now see the *Quick setup* page on GitHub. Copy the code below *push an existing repository from the command line* (Figure 14.4B).

Back in RStudio, paste the code into the **Terminal**. Add your GitHub username and password (important!) (Figure 14.5A). You have now pushed your commit to GitHub, and should be able to see your files in your GitHub account.

The **Pull** and **Push** buttons in RStudio will now also work (Figure 14.5B).

To avoid always having to enter your password, copy the SSH address from GitHub and enter the code shown in Figure 14.5C and D.

Check that the **Pull** and **Push** buttons work as expected (Figure 14.5E). Remember, after each Commit, you have to Push to GitHub, this doesn't happen automatically.

---

[1] It's fine to push some data to GitHub, especially if you want to make it publicly available, but you should do so consciously, not accidentally.

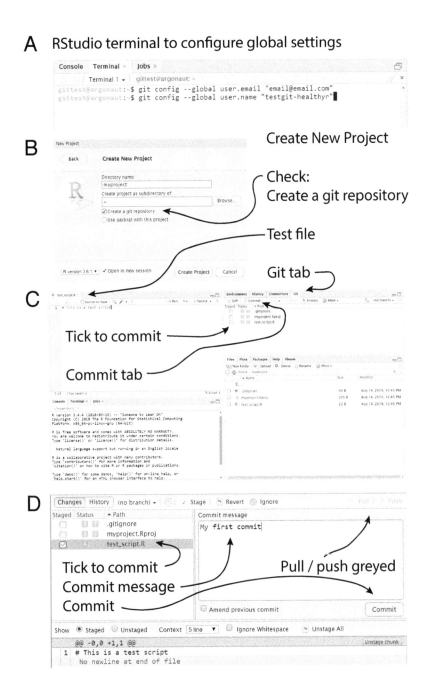

FIGURE 14.3: Configuring your GitHub account via RStudio, creating a new project, commiting a script and pushing it to GitHub.

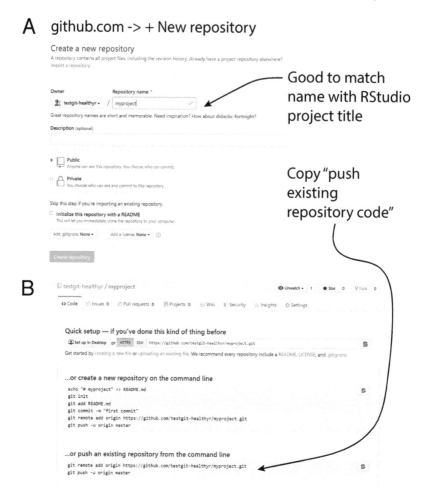

FIGURE 14.4: Create a new repository (repo) on GitHub.

14.5   Clone an existing GitHub project to new RStudio project

An alternative situation is where a project already exists on GitHub and you want to copy it to an RStudio project. In version control world, this is called **cloning**.

In RStudio, click *New project* as normal. Click *Version Control* and select *Git*.

In *Clone Git Repository*, enter the GitHub repository URL as per Figure 14.6C. Change the project directory name if necessary.

As above, to avoid repeatedly having to enter passwords, follow the steps in Figure 14.6D and E.

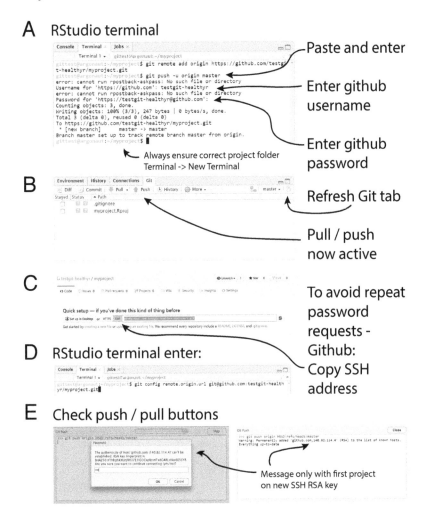

FIGURE 14.5: Linking an RStudio project with a GitHub repository.

14.6 Summary

If your project is worth doing, then it is worth backing up! This means you should use version control for every single project you are involved in. You will quickly be surprised at how many times you wish to go back and rescue some deleted code, or to restore an accidentally deleted file.

It becomes even more important when collaborating and many individuals may be editing the same file. As with the previous chapter, this is an area which data scientists have discovered much later than computer scientists. Get it up and running in your own workflow and you will reap the rewards in the future.

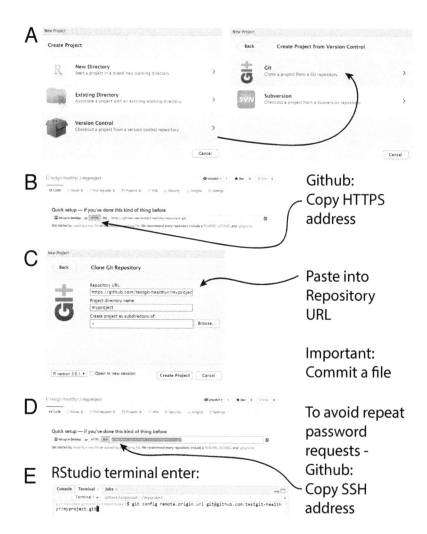

FIGURE 14.6: Clone a GitHub repository to an RStudio project.

15

Encryption

Encryption matters, and it is not just for spies and philanderers.
Glenn Greenwald

Health data is precious and often sensitive. Datasets may contain patient identifiable information. Information may be clearly disclosive, such as a patient's date of birth, post/zip code, or social security number.

Other datasets may have been processed to remove the most obviously confidential information. These still require great care, as the data is usually only 'pseudoanonymised'. This may mean that the data of an individual patient is disclosive when considered as a whole - perhaps the patient had a particularly rare diagnosis. Or it may mean that the data can be combined with other datasets and in combination, individual patients can be identified.

The governance around safe data handling is one of the greatest challenges facing health data scientists today. It needs to be taken very seriously and robust practices must be developed to ensure public confidence.

15.1 Safe practice

Storing sensitive information as raw values leaves the data vulnerable to confidentiality breaches. This is true even when you are working in a 'safe' environment, such as a secure server.

It is best to simply remove as much confidential information from records whenever possible. If the data is not present, then it cannot be compromised.

This might not be a good idea if the data might need to be linked back to an individual at some unspecified point in the future. This may be a problem if, for example, auditors of a clinical trial need to re-identify an individual from the trial data. A study ID can be used, but that still requires the confidential data to be stored and available in a lookup table in another file.

This chapter is not a replacement for an information governance course. These are essential and the reader should follow their institution's guidelines on this. The chapter does introduce a useful R package and encryption functions that you may need to incorporate into your data analysis workflow.

15.2   encryptr package

The **encryptr** package is our own and allows users to store confidential data in a pseudoanonymised form, which is far less likely to result in re-identification.

Either columns in data frames/tibbles or whole files can be directly encrypted from R using strong RSA encryption.

The basis of RSA encryption is a public/private key pair and is the method used of many modern encryption applications. The public key can be shared and is used to encrypt the information.

The private key is sensitive and should not be shared. The private key requires a password to be set, which should follow modern rules on password complexity. You know what you should do! If the password is lost, it cannot be recovered.

15.3   Get the package

The **encryptr** package can be installed in the standard manner or the development version can be obtained from GitHub.

Full documentation is maintained separately at encrypt-r.org[1].

```
install.packages("encryptr")

# Or the development version from Github
remotes::install_github("surgicalinformatics/encryptr")
```

---

[1] https://encrypt-r.org

15.4 Get the data

An example dataset containing the addresses of general practitioners (family doctors) in Scotland is included in the package.

```
library(encryptr)
gp
#> A tibble: 1,212 x 12
#>   organisation_code name    address1 address2 address3 city  postcode
#>   <chr>             <chr>   <chr>    <chr>    <chr>    <chr> <chr>
#> 1 S10002                    MUIRHE... LIFF RO... MUIRHEAD NA     DUND... DD2 5NH
#> 2 S10017                    THE BL... CRIEFF ... KING ST... NA     CRIE... PH7 3SA
```

15.5 Generate private/public keys

The genkeys() function generates a public and private key pair. A password is required to be set in the dialogue box for the private key. Two files are written to the active directory.

The default name for the private key is:

- id_rsa

And for the public key name is generated by default:

- id_rsa.pub

If the private key file is lost, nothing encrypted with the public key can be recovered. Keep this safe and secure. Do not share it without a lot of thought on the implications.

```
genkeys()
#> Private key written with name 'id_rsa'
#> Public key written with name 'id_rsa.pub'
```

15.6   Encrypt columns of data

Once the keys are created, it is possible to encrypt one or more columns of data
in a data frame/tibble using the public key. Every time RSA encryption is used
it will generate a unique output. Even if the same information is encrypted
more than once, the output will always be different. It is therefore not possible
to match two encrypted values.

These outputs are also secure from decryption without the private key. This
may allow sharing of data within or between research teams without sharing
confidential data.

Encrypting columns to a ciphertext is straightforward. However, as stated
above, an important principle is dropping sensitive data which is never going
to be required. Do not hoard more data than you need to answer your question.

```r
library(dplyr)
gp_encrypt = gp %>%
  select(-c(name, address1, address2, address3)) %>%
  encrypt(postcode)
gp_encrypt

#> A tibble: 1,212 x 8
#>   organisation_code city         county      postcode
#>   <chr>             <chr>        <chr>       <chr>
#> 1 S10002            DUNDEE       ANGUS       796284eb46ca…
#> 2 S10017            CRIEFF       PERTHSHIRE  639dfc076ae3…
```

15.7   Decrypt specific information only

Decryption requires the private key generated using `genkeys()` and the password
set at the time. The password and file are not replaceable so need to be kept
safe and secure. It is important to only decrypt the specific pieces of information that are required. The beauty of this system is that when decrypting a
specific cell, the rest of the data remain secure.

```r
gp_encrypt %>%
  slice(1:2) %>%      # Only decrypt the rows and columns necessary
  decrypt(postcode)

#> A tibble: 1,212 x 8
#>   organisation_code city         county      postcode
```

```
#>    <chr>            <chr>       <chr>        <chr>
#> 1 S10002           DUNDEE      ANGUS        DD2 5NH
#> 2 S10017           CRIEFF      PERTHSHIRE  PH7 3SA
```

15.8   Using a lookup table

Rather than storing the ciphertext in the working data frame, a lookup table can be used as an alternative. Using lookup = TRUE has the following effects:

- returns the data frame / tibble with encrypted columns removed and a key column included;
- returns the lookup table as an object in the R environment;
- creates a lookup table .csv file in the active directory.

```
gp_encrypt = gp %>%
  select(-c(name, address1, address2, address3)) %>%
  encrypt(postcode, telephone, lookup = TRUE)

#> Lookup table object created with name 'lookup'
#> Lookup table written to file with name 'lookup.csv'

gp_encrypt

#> A tibble: 1,212 x 7
#>    key   organisation_code city        county      opendate
#>    <int> <chr>             <chr>       <chr>       <date>
#> 1 1      S10002            DUNDEE      ANGUS       1995-05-01
#> 2 2      S10017            CRIEFF      PERTHSHIRE  1996-04-06
```

The file creation can be turned off with write_lookup = FALSE and the name of the lookup can be changed with lookup_name = "anyNameHere". The created lookup file should be itself encrypted using the method below.

Decryption is performed by passing the lookup object or file to the decrypt() function.

```
gp_encrypt %>%
  decrypt(postcode, telephone, lookup_object = lookup)

# Or
gp_encrypt %>%
  decrypt(postcode, telephone, lookup_path = "lookup.csv")

#> A tibble: 1,212 x 8
#>    postcode telephone organisation_code city   county    opendate
#>    <chr>    <chr>     <chr>             <chr>  <chr>     <date>
```

```
#>  1 DD2 5NH 01382 580264 S10002        DUNDEE  ANGUS      1995-05-01
#>  2 PH7 3SA 01764 652283 S10017        CRIEFF  PERTHSHIRE 1996-04-06
```

15.9   Encrypting a file

Encrypting the object within R has little point if a file with the disclosive information is still present on the system. Files can be encrypted and decrypted using the same set of keys.

To demonstrate, the included dataset is written as a .csv file.

```
write_csv(gp, "gp.csv")

encrypt_file("gp.csv")
#> Encrypted file written with name 'gp.csv.encryptr.bin'
```

Check that the file can be decrypted prior to removing the original file from your system.

Warning: it is strongly suggested that the original unencrypted data file backed up in a secure system in case de-encryption is not possible, e.g., the private key file or password is lost.

15.10   Decrypting a file

The decrypt_file function will not allow the original file to be overwritten, therefore use the option to specify a new name for the unencrypted file.

```
decrypt_file("gp.csv.encryptr.bin", file_name = "gp2.csv")

#> Decrypted file written with name 'gp2.csv'
```

15.11 Ciphertexts are not matchable

The ciphertext produced for a given input will change with each encryption. This is a feature of the RSA algorithm. Ciphertexts should not therefore be attempted to be matched between datasets encrypted using the same public key. This is a conscious decision given the risks associated with sharing the necessary details.

15.12 Providing a public key

In collaborative projects where data may be pooled, a public key can be made available by you via a link to enable collaborators to encrypt sensitive data. This provides a robust method for sharing potentially disclosive data points.

```
gp_encrypt = gp %>%
  select(-c(name, address1, address2, address3)) %>%
  encrypt(postcode, telephone, public_key_path =
            "https://argonaut.is.ed.ac.uk/public/id_rsa.pub")
```

15.13 Use cases

15.13.1 Blinding in trials

A potential application is maintaining blinding / allocation concealment in randomised controlled clinical trials. Using the same method of encryption, it is possible to encrypt the participant allocation group, allowing the sharing of data without compromising blinding. If other members of the trial team are permitted to see treatment allocation (unblinded), then the decryption process can be followed to reveal the group allocation.

The benefit of this approach is that each ciphertext is unique. This prevents researchers identifying patterns of outcomes or adverse events within a named group such as "Group A". Instead, each participant appears to have a truly unique allocation group which can only be revealed by the decryption process. In situations such as block randomisation, where the trial enrolment personnel are blinded to the allocation, this unique ciphertext further limits the impact of selection bias.

15.13.2   Re-contacting participants

Clinical research often requires further contact of participants for either planned follow-up or sometimes in cases of early cessation of trials due to harm. **encryptr** allows the storage of contact details in pseudoanonymised format that can be decrypted only when necessary.

For example, investigators running a randomised clinical trial of a novel therapeutic agent may decide that all enrolled participants taking another medication should withdraw due to a major drug interaction. Using a basic filter, patients taking this medication could be identified and the telephone numbers decrypted for these participants. The remaining telephone numbers would remain encrypted preventing unnecessary re-identification of participants.

15.13.3   Long-term follow-up of participants

Researchers with approved projects may one day receive approval to carry out additional follow-up through tracking of outcomes through electronic healthcare records or re-contact of patients. Should a follow-up study be approved, patient identifiers stored as ciphertexts could then be decrypted to allow matching of the participant to their own health records.

15.14   Summary

All confidential information must be treated with the utmost care. Data should never be carried on removable devices or portable computers. Data should never be sent by open email. Encrypting data provides some protection against disclosure. But particularly in healthcare, data often remains potentially disclosive (or only pseudoanonymised) even after encryption of identifiable variables. Treat it with great care and respect.

Appendix

This book was written in **bookdown**, which is an R package built on top of R Markdown (Xie (2016)).

The main packages used in this book were: **tidyverse, ggplot2, tibble, tidyr, readr, purrr, dplyr, stringr, forcats, finalfit, bookdown, broom, encryptr, gapminder, GGally, ggfortify, kableExtra, knitr, lme4, lubridate, magrittr, mice, MissMech, patchwork, rmarkdown, scales, survival, and survminer**.

R and package versions, `sessionInfo()`:

```
## R version 3.6.1 (2019-07-05)
## Platform: x86_64-pc-linux-gnu (64-bit)
## Running under: Ubuntu 16.04.6 LTS
##
## Locale:
##    LC_CTYPE=en_GB.UTF-8       LC_NUMERIC=C
##    LC_TIME=en_GB.UTF-8        LC_COLLATE=en_GB.UTF-8
##    LC_MONETARY=en_GB.UTF-8    LC_MESSAGES=en_GB.UTF-8
##    LC_PAPER=en_GB.UTF-8       LC_NAME=C
##    LC_ADDRESS=C               LC_TELEPHONE=C
##    LC_MEASUREMENT=en_GB.UTF-8 LC_IDENTIFICATION=C
##
## Package version:
##    bookdown_0.20.2     broom_0.7.0         dplyr_1.0.0
##    encryptr_0.1.3      finalfit_1.0.2      forcats_0.5.0
##    gapminder_0.3.0     GGally_2.0.0        ggfortify_0.4.10
##    ggplot2_3.3.2       kableExtra_1.1.0.9000 knitr_1.29
##    lme4_1.1.23         lubridate_1.7.9     magrittr_1.5
##    mice_3.10.0         MissMech_1.0.2      patchwork_1.0.1
##    purrr_0.3.4         readr_1.3.1         rmarkdown_2.3
##    scales_1.1.1        stringr_1.4.0       survival_3.2.3
##    survminer_0.4.7     tibble_3.0.3        tidyr_1.1.0
##    tidyverse_1.3.0
```

Bibliography

Bryan, J. (2017). *gapminder: Data from Gapminder.* R package version 0.3.0.

Harrell, F. (2015). *Regression Modeling Strategies: With Applications to Linear Models, Logistic and Ordinal Regression, and Survival Analysis.* Springer Series in Statistics. Springer International Publishing, 2 edition.

Harrower, M. and Brewer, C. A. (2003). Colorbrewer.org: An online tool for selecting colour schemes for maps. *The Cartographic Journal*, 40(1):27–37.

Terry M. Therneau and Patricia M. Grambsch (2000). *Modeling Survival Data: Extending the Cox Model.* Springer, New York.

Therneau, T. M. (2020). *A Package for Survival Analysis in R.* R package version 3.2-3.

Wickham, H. (2016). *ggplot2: Elegant Graphics for Data Analysis.* Springer-Verlag New York.

Wickham, H., Averick, M., Bryan, J., Chang, W., McGowan, L., François, R., Grolemund, G., Hayes, A., Henry, L., Hester, J., Kuhn, M., Pedersen, T., Miller, E., Bache, S., Müller, K., Ooms, J., Robinson, D., Seidel, D., Spinu, V., Takahashi, K., Vaughan, D., Wilke, C., Woo, K., and Yutani, H. (2019). Welcome to the tidyverse. *Journal of Open Source Software*, 4(43):1686.

Xie, Y. (2016). *bookdown: Authoring Books and Technical Documents with R Markdown.* Chapman and Hall/CRC. ISBN 978-1138700109.

Index

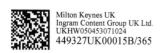

9 780367 428198